D1715218

Allies and Adversaries

The Impact of Managed Care on Mental Health Services

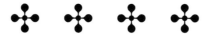

Allies and Adversaries

The Impact of Managed Care on Mental Health Services

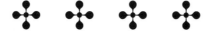

EDITED BY
Robert K. Schreter, M.D.
Steven S. Sharfstein, M.D., M.P.A.
Carol A. Schreter, M.S.W., Ph.D.

American Psychiatric Press, Inc.
Washington, DC
London, England

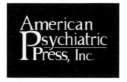

Note: The authors have worked to ensure that all information in this book concerning drug dosages, schedules, and routes of administration is accurate as of the time of publication and consistent with standards set by the U.S. Food and Drug Administration and the general medical community. As medical research and practice advance, however, therapeutic standards may change. For this reason and because human and mechanical errors sometimes occur, we recommend that readers follow the advice of a physician who is directly involved in their care or the care of a member of their family.

Copyright © 1994 American Psychiatric Press
ALL RIGHTS RESERVED
Manufactured in the United States of America on acid-free paper
97 96 95 94   4 3 2 1
First Edition

American Psychiatric Press, Inc.
1400 K Street, N.W., Washington, DC   20005

Library of Congress Cataloging-in-Publication Data
Allies and adversaries : the impact of managed care on mental health services /
edited by Robert K. Schreter, Steven S. Sharfstein, Carol A. Schreter.
    p.   cm.
    Includes bibliographical references and index.
    ISBN (invalid) 0-88048-667-5 (alk. paper)
    1. Managed mental health care—United States.   I. Schreter, Robert
K., 1945- . II. Sharfstein, Steven S. (Steven Samuel), 1942- . III.
Schreter, Carol A., 1947- .
    [DNLM: 1. Managed Care Programs—United States. 2. Mental
Health Services—United States.   W 275 AA1 A43 1994]
  RC465.6.A39   1994
  362.2'0973—dc20
  DNLM/DLC   94-368
  for Library of Congress   CIP

British Library Cataloguing in Publication Data
A CIP record is available from the British Library.

Contents

Contributors   ix

Preface   xiii

Section I: A Corporate Perspective

✛ CHAPTER 1 ✛

From Fee-for-Service to Accountable Health Plans   3
   Mary Jane England, M.D.

Section II: Clinical Services

✛ CHAPTER 2 ✛

Inpatient Services   11

   The Managed Care View—*Henry T. Harbin, M.D.*

   The Clinician's View—*Glen O. Gabbard, M.D.*

✛ CHAPTER 3 ✛

Intermediate Levels of Care   31

   The Managed Care View—*Kenneth A. Kessler, M.D.*

   The Clinician's View—*Richard D. Budson, M.D.*

✛ CHAPTER 4 ✛

Outpatient Services   51

   The Managed Care View—*Daniel Y. Patterson, M.D., M.P.H.*

   The Clinician's View—*Robert K. Schreter, M.D.*

✛ CHAPTER 5 ✛

Child and Adolescent Services   69

   The Managed Care View—*Ronald Geraty, M.D.*

   The Clinician's View—*Alan A. Axelson, M.D.*

✣ CHAPTER 6 ✣

Drugs and Alcohol   85

The Managed Care View—*Chip Silverman, Ph.D., M.P.H.*

The Clinician's View—*Sheldon I. Miller, M.D.*

Section III: Providers of Clinical Services

✣ CHAPTER 7 ✣

The Role of the Psychiatrist   103

The Managed Care View—*Anthony F. Panzetta, M.D.*

The Clinician's View—*Joanne H. Ritvo, M.D.*

✣ CHAPTER 8 ✣

The Role of the Psychologist   117

The Managed Care View—*Nicholas A. Cummings, Ph.D., Litt.D.*

The Clinician's View—*Daniel J. Abrahamson, Ph.D.,
and Alfred A. Lucco, Ph.D.*

✣ CHAPTER 9 ✣

The Role of the Social Worker   135

The Managed Care View—*Norman Winegar, A.C.S.W., L.C.S.W*

The Clinician's View—*Mary Jo Monahan, L.C.S.W.*

Section IV: Emerging Clinical Issues

✣ CHAPTER 10 ✣

Practice Guidelines   153

The Managed Care View—*John Bartlett, M.D., M.P.H.*

The Clinician's View—*John S. McIntyre, M.D.*

✣ CHAPTER 11 ✣

Quality-of-Care Guidelines   169

 The Managed Care View—*Alex R. Rodriguez, M.D.*

 The Clinician's View—*Robert W. Gibson, M.D.*

✣ CHAPTER 12 ✣

Ethical Issues Under Managed Care   187

 The Managed Care View—*James E. Sabin, M.D.*

 The Clinician's View—*Steven S. Sharfstein, M.D., M.P.A.*

Section V: A Family Perspective

✣ CHAPTER 13 ✣

Managed Care and Mental Illness   203
 Laurie M. Flynn, National Alliance for the Mentally Ill (NAMI)

Section VI: Managing Care, Not Dollars

✣ CHAPTER 14 ✣

How Adversaries Can Become Allies   213
 Robert K. Schreter, M.D.
 Steven S. Sharfstein, M.D., M.P.A.
 Carol A. Schreter, M.S.W., Ph.D.

Index   221

Contributors

Daniel J. Abrahamson, Ph.D.
Administrative Director, The Traumatic Stress Institute, South Windsor, Connecticut; State and Federal Advocacy Coordinator, Connecticut Psychological Association; Consultant, American Psychological Association—Practice Directorate

Alan A. Axelson, M.D.
Medical Director and Chief Executive Officer, InterCare–Comprehensive Behavioral Healthcare, Pittsburgh, Pennsylvania; Chairman, Work Group on Managed Care, American Academy of Child and Adolescent Psychiatry

John Bartlett, M.D., M.P.H.
Vice President and Corporate Medical Director, MCC Behavioral Care, Eden Prairie, Minnesota

Richard D. Budson, M.D.
Assistant General Director, McLean Hospital, Belmont, Massachusetts; Director, Community Residential and Treatment Program, McLean Hospital, Belmont, Massachusetts; Associate Professor of Psychiatry, Harvard Medical School, Boston, Massachusetts

Nicholas A. Cummings, Ph.D., Litt.D.
President, Foundation for Behavioral Health, San Francisco, California; founding Chairman and Chief Executive Officer, American Biodyne (retired), San Francisco, California; President, National Academies of Practice; former President, American Psychological Association

Mary Jane England, M.D.
President, Washington Business Group on Health, Washington, DC; National Program Director, Mental Health Services for Youth, Robert Wood Johnson Foundation, Princeton, New Jersey; Treasurer of the American Psychiatric Association, Washington, DC

Laurie M. Flynn
Executive Director of the National Alliance for the Mentally Ill (NAMI), based in Arlington, Virginia (NAMI is a national grassroots family and consumer organization advocating on behalf of persons with severe psychiatric disorders.)

Glen O. Gabbard, M.D.
Director, C. F. Menninger Memorial Hospital, and Vice President for Adult Services, The Menninger Clinic, Topeka, Kansas; Clinical Professor of Psychiatry, University of Kansas School of Medicine, Kansas City, Kansas

Ronald Geraty, M.D.
Executive Vice President of Medco Behavioral Care Corporation, Burlington, Massachusetts; Instructor in Psychiatry, Department of Psychiatry, Harvard Medical School at the Cambridge Hospital, Cambridge, Massachusetts

Robert W. Gibson, M.D.
President Emeritus, The Sheppard and Enoch Pratt Hospital, Baltimore, Maryland

Henry T. Harbin, M.D.
President and Chief Executive Officer, Green Spring Health Services, Inc., Columbia, Maryland; Clinical Professor of Psychiatry, University of Maryland School of Medicine, Baltimore, Maryland

Kenneth A. Kessler, M.D.
Founder and President of American Psych Systems, Bethesda, Maryland; founder and former Chief Executive Officer of American PsychManagement, Rosslyn, Virginia

Alfred A. Lucco, Ph.D.
Cofounder, The Center for Development (a multispecialty mental health group), Baltimore, Maryland; Associate Professor, School of Social Work, University of Maryland at Baltimore

John S. McIntyre, M.D.
President, American Psychiatric Association; private practice in psychiatry, Rochester, New York; Chair, Department of Psychiatry, St. Mary's Hospital, Rochester, New York; and Clinical Professor of Psychiatry, University of Rochester, Rochester, New York

Sheldon I. Miller, M.D.
Director, Stone Institute of Psychiatry, Northwestern Memorial Hospital, Chicago, Illinois; Lizzie Gilman Professor and Chair, Department of Psychiatry and Behavioral Sciences, Northwestern University Medical School, Chicago, Illinois

Mary Jo Monahan, L.C.S.W.
Clinical social worker in private practice, associated with Psychotherapy and Employee Assistance Consultants, Tampa, Florida; Chairperson, Competence Certification Commission, National Association of Social Workers; Adjunct Professor in School of Social Work, University of South Florida, Tampa, Florida

Anthony F. Panzetta, M.D.
President and Chief Executive Officer, TAO, Inc., Philadelphia, Pennsylvania; former Professor and Chairman of the Department of Psychiatry, Temple University Medical School, Philadelphia, Pennsylvania

Daniel Y. Patterson, M.D., M.P.H.
Private practice in psychiatry, Wilmington, North Carolina; managed care consultant

Joanne H. Ritvo, M.D.
Private practice in psychiatry, Denver, Colorado; Associate Clinical Professor of Psychiatry, University of Colorado Health Sciences Center, Denver, Colorado; Consultant, American Psychiatric Association Managed Care Committee; former Medical Director, Adult Unit, West Pines Psychiatric Hospital, Wheatridge, Colorado

Alex R. Rodriguez, M.D.
Chief Medical Officer, Preferred Works/Value Health, Wilton, Connecticut; Instructor in Psychiatry, Yale University School of Medicine, New Haven, Connecticut

James E. Sabin, M.D.
Associate Director, Teaching Programs, Harvard Community Health Plan; Assistant Clinical Professor of Psychiatry, Harvard Medical School, Boston, Massachusetts

Carol A. Schreter, M.S.W., Ph.D.
Authors' editor and freelance writer on health and aging, based in Baltimore, Maryland

Robert K. Schreter, M.D.
Private practice in psychiatry, Baltimore, Maryland; Medical Director, Psych Services, Baltimore, Maryland; Assistant Professor of Psychiatry, Johns Hopkins Medical School, Baltimore, Maryland

Steven S. Sharfstein, M.D., M.P.A.

Medical Director and Chief Executive Officer, The Sheppard and Enoch Pratt Hospital, Baltimore, Maryland; Clinical Professor of Psychiatry, University of Maryland Medical School, Baltimore, Maryland

Chip Silverman, Ph.D., M.P.H.

Director of Chemical Dependency, Government Relations and Public Affairs, Green Spring Health Services, Inc., Columbia, Maryland; former director of the Maryland Alcohol and Drug Abuse Administration

Norman Winegar, A.C.S.W., L.C.S.W.

Executive Director of MCC Behavioral Care, Richmond, Virginia; clinical administrator in managed care settings

Preface

Managed care is the inevitable consequence of forces that have been building over the past half century. This era is only part of a long process of change.

Mental health services have unfolded in three distinct periods since 1940. Buoyed by the success of World War II battlefield interventions, psychiatry was legitimized and psychotherapy was popularized in the 1940s and 1950s. Between 1960 and 1980, the nation's commitment to mental health spurred the Community Mental Health Center movement. The number and types of mental health providers exploded. These expansions occurred without regard to the cost of the services provided.

However, the period since 1980 has been dominated by concern about effectiveness and efficiency. Government sags under the burden of its health care expenditures. Industry struggles with the cost of medical care for employees, a cost equal to corporate after-tax profits. Managed care emerged as an effort to introduce cost as a crucial element in clinical decision making and health care policy. Managed care involves accountability for every dollar spent. It has led to providers joining immense, cost-conscious networks.

The evolution of managed care has been associated with distress and distrust. On the one side are clinicians—psychiatrists, psychologists, psychiatric nurses, and social workers—who feel they know what their patients need, especially with regard to quality and quantity. Clinicians often view the efforts of cost regulators as a malignant intrusion, threatening patient and clinician alike. On the other side is an industry whose product is cost savings to those who pay for the care. Industry spokespeople talk about the practice of psychiatry as a cottage industry and speak of abuses in the system, both naive and intended.

In the space between the clinicians' and reviewers' points of view, a structure is emerging. This structure is flawed. It can be improved. A better system is needed as government moves toward ensuring mental health coverage for all Americans.

We believe that mental health providers need to understand the forces at work—if they are to help develop treatment strategies and systems that address the needs of consumers, payers, and clinicians. Overall, in health care, the tensions between providers and cost reviewers will persist, no matter who pays for the care. American citizens expect more, and providers will suggest more, than even national health insurance can afford.

In an era of limited resources, this book presents a platform for the seemingly polar positions of providers and cost reviewers. In nearly every chapter, a prominent representative of each community speaks. First a managed care executive shares his or her expectations and frustrations. Then a clinician does the same. Of special interest, placed just before the editors' conclusion, is a critique of managed care by the National Alliance for the Mentally Ill, from the important perspective of patients and families.

For this book, 26 industry leaders—mostly clinicians and managed care executives—responded to a set of questions in early 1993. Essentially, each was asked two questions, both from the viewpoint of clinical care: 1) What do you believe are the major problems with managed mental health care? 2) What would you do to improve the situation? The reader will not find here a scholarly, objective voice. Instead, these essays reflect the personal beliefs and passions of mental health industry leaders.

This juxtaposition of views is offered in the spirit of promoting dialogue. This is not a how-to book with easy answers. But you may be surprised, as we were, to sense a convergence of views, especially regarding the major problem areas. In these pages, three communities—clinicians, cost reviewers, and family members—share the search for accessible, effective, affordable mental health care systems.

The Editors

Section I

A Corporate Perspective

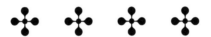

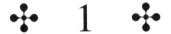

1

From Fee-for-Service to Accountable Health Plans

MARY JANE ENGLAND, M.D.[*]

The American health care system is fragmented, expensive, and unfair. In 1992, health care costs in the United States had spiraled to 14% of the gross national product—approximately $840 billion dollars, an increase from the prior year of more than 13%. The average per-employee cost in the United States for large employers was $3,900, according to Foster Higgins. The United States spends more money per capita than any other country in the world, and yet the system is unfair to many Americans. Thirty-seven million Americans are uninsured; of that number, 11 million are children. According to the Employee Benefit Research Institute, in 1992 approximately 60 million Americans were underinsured for health care. This situation was a particular concern for patients with mental health and substance abuse problems, because many of them had used up their limited benefits or run out of their lifetime maximum coverage for mental health.

Mental health system reform is an important part of health system reform. Throughout the last 10 years, mental health care costs have risen faster than health care cost increases, particularly in the private-sector

[*]President, Washington Business Group on Health, Washington, DC; National Program Director, Mental Health Services for Youth, Robert Wood Johnson Foundation, Princeton, New Jersey; Treasurer of the American Psychiatric Association, Washington, DC.

coverage of mental health and substance abuse. Much of this increase was due to poor benefit design. A design of 45 days of inpatient treatment and 20 days of outpatient treatment at 50% copayment led to inappropriate and unnecessary care in costly inpatient settings. Abuse of the 45-day inpatient hospitalization benefit was seen, particularly in the areas of adolescent hospitalization and substance abuse treatment. We saw the dramatic growth of 28-day substance abuse treatment programs and prolonged hospitalization programs for adolescents. The benefit did not provide for flexibility or allow for appropriate ambulatory or less-intensive treatment for these disorders. This benefit plan was designed as a way to protect those most in need of mental health services. However, the practice discouraged early intervention and less restrictive coverage. Furthermore, the scope of services often covered by traditional benefit plans was limited to just inpatient and outpatient treatment. There was no flexibility for intermediary services such as partial hospital, residential, day, and evening treatment programs and in-home family counseling.

Service delivery remains fragmented in the mental health system and is similar to that in the medical system. Utilization review of a large company revealed that two of three individuals who were hospitalized for mental health services did not receive follow-up ambulatory care. Case management is unavailable in traditional indemnity plans. Another problem with the current mental health delivery system is the poor recognition and treatment of mental illness and substance abuse problems in primary care settings. A study done by the Rand Corporation stated that primary care physicians detected depression in only 51% of patients with a current depressive disorder receiving fee-for-service care.

The development of managed mental health in the mid-1980s was a laudable effort by insurers and businesses to curb costs and improve quality. Employers want a healthy, productive work force at a cost they can afford. Both public and private employers provide subsidized health insurance as well as subsidized health and disability insurance for their employees.

The first generation of managed care, starting in 1984, involved utilization review alone. This process was purely one of administrative oversight. In order for the insurer to pay for a mental health service, the care had to be preauthorized. Nurses, often supervised by surgeons, were hired to make such decisions on a case-by-case basis. Unfortunately, adversarial relations with providers developed quickly, in great part because reviewers were not knowledgeable about mental illness. Soon insurers and managed care companies began hiring reviewers with more appropriate training—psychiatric social workers and nurses supervised by psychiatrists.

This first generation was moderately successful in decreasing the inappropriate use of in-hospital care. However, benefits remained capped. This benefit cap failed to address the underlying problem of bad benefit design. It still left patients without access to preventive and ambulatory care.

The second generation of managed mental health care, starting in 1990, might be called "utilization review with selected providers." Managed care companies developed networks of providers, including psychiatrists, psychologists, and psychiatric social workers. Therapists were selected in terms of quality and because they accepted the idea of cost-conscious, effective care. Patient referrals were limited to these preferred providers.

To address the issue of bad benefit design, some managed care companies offered to pay for services along a continuum of care, often including partial hospitalization, supervised group living situations, and intensive in-home service. Contracted providers were given authority and flexibility to shift patients to these more appropriate levels of care. Decision making was returned to the provider.

However, benefits were still limited, capped in terms of dollars allowed per patient per year. Too many mentally ill people and substance abusers reached these limits and found themselves without mental health insurance.

The Carve-Out Contract

Employers began to separate ("carve out") mental health and substance abuse care from major medical benefits, buying this care from another vendor promising to offer better cost and quality controls. With carve outs, instead of limiting benefits per person, employers pool the risks for their employee group. Employers pay a fixed per-capita rate for all covered workers and dependents. A large employer, for example, might have 12,000 employees in an area. With dependents, this group might total 28,000. Carve-out companies bidding for this contract must make assumptions about the demand. It might be assumed, for instance, that in any month, 8% of the covered population will ask for mental health services.

This kind of contract, with a flat per-person fee, allows providers to make decisions about services provided. The provider is at risk financially for cost overruns. If the carve-out company spends more than the allocated cost per person, the company suffers the loss. A range of services is available, so that the most appropriate service is most likely to be used. Such a system might include outpatient therapy, intensive in-home services, respite care, partial hospitalization, and group homes, as well as both short- and long-term inpatient care.

Five companies begun in the era of utilization review have grown with each of these changes. They survive as the major carve-out companies: American Psych Management, U.S. Behavioral Health, Preferred Health, Biodyne, and Managed Health Networks. At this point, they and smaller competitors are bidding at wildly different rates and offering employers different combinations of services.

Underbidding is a problem with some of the carve-out contracts being signed today. Theoretically, underbidding cuts provider profits, but it also leads to cost cutting in the form of denying care to patients who would otherwise receive it.

All of this change in systems and financing has occurred since 1990. What is perhaps most surprising, however, is not the pace of the change but the scope. It is not something happening on the periphery of medicine. By 1992, an estimated 75% of employees (and their dependents) at moderate-size to large American businesses were enrolled in managed mental health care systems. This percentage is high even compared with that for medical and surgical care, for which 50% of workers and their dependents use managed care systems.

The Need for Paradigm Shifts

Accountability—Cost, Quality, and Outcomes

Because of rising costs, purchasers of care tend to scrutinize medicine more closely. Payers and consumers want to understand what works in medicine so that only appropriate care is delivered and reimbursed.

In purchasing health care services, payers want to know whether, with this care, the consumer will maintain health, go back to work or school, and function better at home or in the community. Purchasers are demanding such functional outcome measures from all providers of health care services.

For mental health providers, the great challenge now is to appreciate the importance of using functional outcome measures. We must be able to measure the impact of the care we provide. The price that employers will pay depends on what they expect to get for their dollars. The routine use of such measures will help mental health to get back into the mainstream of medicine.

Fortunately, mental health services research has made great progress since 1990. Tools are now available to measure outcomes for the treatment of depression, anxiety, alcohol abuse, and—soon—schizophrenia.

Intuitively, mental health providers recognize the good they are doing. However, we have not yet focused enough energy on showing payers that we are effective. We must certainly work harder at this task, probably harder than other disciplines because we share the stigma that is attached to our patients.

The Future: Accountable Health Plans

The language of this book is probably already outdated. The term *managed care* has been replaced, in the minds of many, by the term *managed competition*. The phrase *systems of care* has been replaced by the terms *organized systems of care* or *accountable health plans*.

A system of care is accountable to payers and to patients. Patients now form an identifiable purchasing group. Are the systems we now have of the quality we want them to be? Decidedly not!

The basics of a good system include the following:

✢ Access for all Americans
✢ Full entitlement for mentally ill and substance-abusing persons
✢ Integrated financing and delivery systems with a continuum of services
✢ Payment for services linked to the performance of the system of care

Full entitlement means the availability of preventive, primary, acute, rehabilitative, and chronic care. Arbitrary benefit limits are not necessary. The goal of care is to maximize the patient's functional capacity.

Payment is linked to the performance of the system, not to the performance of the individual patient or even the provider. Providers will fail to help some patients, of course. This inevitability must be built in to the cost of care.

To pay for such expanded care for all Americans, employers could pay 75% for the standard benefit. Workers could pay 25%. Households with an income below 200% of the poverty line could get government help with the cost of premiums, on a sliding fee scale.

To prevent underbidding on contracts and then denying needed care, an accountable health plan could be required to meet national standards set by a national health board. In mental health care, such standards might require the following:

❖ A 24-hour capacity to address crises
❖ The ability to respond within 3 days to regular calls for help
❖ The ability to respond within hours for emergencies
❖ A minimum number and variety of providers
❖ A continuum of care

A national health board could set standards for the composition of the mental health team, based on the size and demographics of the population served. These standards might include the proportions of psychiatrists, psychologists, and psychiatric social workers. Standards might also require that therapists come from diverse cultures and have age-appropriate training (i.e., training in child and adolescent or elderly psychiatry). Licensed providers at the state level might refine such measures—for example, by deciding whether a system should include providers with foreign-language skills.

To summarize, this has been a tumultuous decade for mental health care. Inappropriate and unnecessary utilization of a badly designed, limited mental health benefit has led to no scientific evidence to support limited-benefit designs. We must focus on necessary and appropriate mental health and substance abuse treatment in the context of an "accountable mental health plan."

Section II

Clinical Services

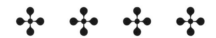

❖ 2 ❖

Inpatient Services

The Managed Care View

HENRY T. HARBIN, M.D.[*]

The conflicts and controversies between managed care companies and psychiatric hospitals have been bitter and protracted. The accusations of unethical and/or inappropriate interventions by managed care companies against psychiatric hospitals and by psychiatric hospitals against managed care companies have damaged the reputations of both. The intensity of the struggle may have been a necessary developmental step in the process of bringing about changes in hospital practice patterns. But the issues have been polarized beyond any factual parameters. There now appear to be increasing degrees of collaboration between inpatient providers and managed care mental health and substance abuse companies that will hopefully lead to a more constructive clinical reality for patients who need this type of care.

In this chapter, I outline the factors that contributed to the polarization and the changes that have been made by inpatient providers and managed

[*]President and Chief Executive Officer, Green Spring Health Services, Inc., Columbia, Maryland; Clinical Professor of Psychiatry, University of Maryland School of Medicine, Baltimore, Maryland.

care companies. These changes have led to some positive trends that
should produce constructive alliances in the future between the hospital
industry and managed care programs.

Contributions by Hospitals
to the Problem of Cost Versus Quality

Many psychiatric and substance abuse inpatient programs have continued or developed practices over the past 15 years that have increased
costs unnecessarily, limited quality care, and invited insurance companies and managed care programs to intervene aggressively with their cost
containment programs. I want to qualify that statement by noting that the
trends identified in this chapter were not followed or set by all hospitals.
Many inpatient providers have provided cost-effective, high-quality care
for decades and have consequently had to make minimal modifications
in this era of managed care.

Excess Hospital Bed Capacity

During the 1970s and early 1980s, the psychiatric and substance abuse
industry overexpanded the needed number of beds in many parts of the
country. The causes of this overexpansion were severalfold: 1) the expansion of for-profit hospital chains into psychiatric and substance abuse
care, 2) the reduction in regulatory oversight in many states (i.e., the
abolishment of "certificate of need" requirements), 3) the expansion of
insurance benefits to cover substance abuse and psychiatric care, and 4)
the passage of state mandates requiring minimum benefits for mental
health and substance abuse care. The more aggressive market-oriented
hospitals provided beds beyond the needed capacity, leading to increased
competition for occupancy and to increased lengths of stay. In some
parts of the country, psychiatric and substance abuse hospitals were routinely operating at 40%–60% capacity due to the excess number of beds.

Overreliance on Inpatient Care as the Preferred
Treatment Modality

Many hospital providers and outpatient professionals had become overly
dependent on hospital care to handle difficult patients. This trend was

encouraged by the tendency of insurance companies to limit outpatient benefits while providing 100% coverage for inpatient care. The malpractice litigation crisis of the 1970s and 1980s fueled this trend, because hospitalizing a patient was frequently the safest (and easiest) alternative and certainly the least risky from a legal perspective. The substance abuse inpatient industry was particularly at fault in this area. During the 1980s, the prominent view was that anyone with a moderate to serious chemical dependence problem needed inpatient care before receiving any other type of care. A rigid philosophy of care developed in the substance abuse community that promoted inpatient treatment as the only acceptable intervention. This philosophy of treatment was exploited by some for-profit chains that realized that these programs were extremely profitable.

Fixed Lengths of Stay

Many, but not all, hospital programs tended to keep patients until all inpatient insurance benefits were exhausted. Frequently, hospital records would reflect patients as dangerous and suicidal until the last day of the benefit limit, and then the patient would be miraculously cured. Many substance abuse programs continue these practices today. The lack of individualized care for inpatients created a significant credibility problem for the hospital industry with insurance companies and the public. Many inpatient providers were unwilling to provide flexible lengths of stay. Patients were placed into ward programs that were not tailored to their individual needs (e.g., family visits were always held in the third week of the inpatient stay or leaves of absence were reserved only for weekends). Again, the "28-day" substance abuse inpatient programs were notorious for having rigid programming that was not specific to the individual nature of the problems.

Profit Motive

Psychiatric and substance abuse hospitals have made a great deal of money over the past 15 years. As margins were squeezed by cost containment in the medical and surgical areas, many general hospitals expanded their mental health and substance abuse units. It must be remembered that most psychiatric programs were exempt from the Medicare diagnosis-related group program, and this exemption led to significant cost shifting by the hospital industry. With the advent of managed mental health and substance abuse programs, these profit margins have been squeezed, leading to the elimination of beds or the closure of whole facilities. Many hospitals have responded by keeping patients longer or admitting patients unnecessarily in order to maintain their profit margins. Many psychiatrists were motivated to admit and keep patients longer because the professional reimbursement was often better in an inpatient setting. Again, the insurance companies have encouraged this trend. A psychiatrist could receive 80%–100% reimbursement at a higher rate for inpatient services but receive only 50%–60% reimbursement at a lower rate for outpatient care for the same patient. Consequently, a psychiatrist could bill from five to seven professional visits per week for an inpatient at 80% coverage, whereas the same person might be billed only once or twice per week as an outpatient at 50% coverage. The fiscal incentives were clearly in place to encourage overutilization of inpatient services.

Fraud and Abuse in the Hospital Industry

Although there have been some clearly documented examples of unethical billing practices and fraud, I believe that these have been the exceptions. Some for-profit chains have established bonus schemes to recruit patients and to reward professionals inappropriately for hospitalized patients. Fraudulent billing practices have also been discovered. These extremes have provided justifications for insurance companies and managed care programs to take action.

Delays in Technology Transmission

It is interesting to note that the public sector was far ahead of the private sector in developing innovative alternatives to hospital care. These services were often provided to the poorest patients and financed by state and federal governments. Many research studies in the 1970s and 1980s documented that seriously ill patients could be managed effectively outside of hospitals. Yet this technology was not generalized to many private hospitals, clearly in part because of the economic incentives described previously. Many inpatient practitioners who were not motivated by financial factors continued their philosophy of treatment that inpatient care was superior or the only way to treat many patients. This phenomenon has been particularly present with substance abuse inpatient programs, which in the 1980s had an especially difficult time responding to scientific data and the need for more flexible treatment patterns.

Problems in the Managed Care Industry

Many, but not all, managed care companies have introduced practices that have been detrimental to collaborative relationships with hospitals. Like the above-mentioned hospital trends, these practices were more prevalent during the 1980s and in the early stages of the managed mental health care movement, whereas more constructive changes have been seen in the past several years. Some managed care companies have had a philosophy of being overtly hostile to inpatient care of any kind and have adopted an antihospital attitude. Although some of their practices were clearly successful in cutting costs, the consequence was often reduction of access and poor-quality care. These excessive practices have also given a "black eye" to the managed care industry.

Secret Criteria

Review criteria and appeals procedures were (and still are in some companies) often secret and proprietary. The secret criteria left clinicians uncertain as to how to offer an accurate, complete, and relevant response to requests for information. The lack of public criteria encouraged arbitrary and inconsistent review decisions by managed care companies. Hospital stays could be denied based on criteria that would not be shared with the provider, leaving both the patient and the provider angry and frustrated in their interactions with managed care companies.

Inappropriate Credentials of Review Personnel

The qualifications of review staff who evaluated and challenged critical medical and psychiatric decisions were often vague or inappropriate. Many firms did not have specialty mental health or substance abuse staff conducting reviews, and those that did rarely had psychiatrists involved in an integral, primary manner. First-generation utilization review firms usually had medical-surgical nurses and primary care physicians conducting psychiatric reviews. At times, nonphysician staff would deny inpatient care without a clear independent appeals process.

Excessive Administrative Time

Utilization review activities often presented an increased administrative burden for providers. This burden was worsened when reviewers were not readily accessible. Many managed care firms did not have 24-hour availability or had physician reviewers who were unavailable after care had been denied. Frequently, managed care companies would have different reviewers manage the same case from review to review so that the provider had to represent the cases frequently.

Excessive Cost Cutting

Some managed care firms inappropriately rewarded reviewers to deny care and or went too far in denying needed hospital care. A few psychiatric managed care firms were proud of the fact that they had between 1 and 5 hospital days per 1,000 patients, reflecting inappropriately low utilization of inpatient services. Typically, the only way such low levels of utilization could be reached involved denials of access and/or limiting benefits for seriously ill patients.

Health Maintenance Organization Restrictions on Chronic Patients

Many of the flagrant abuses of managed care programs have been in health maintenance organizations (HMOs). Many HMO gatekeepers, especially those not in the mental health field, have severely limited outpatient care for mental health and substance abuse. Typically, HMO mental health and substance abuse benefits have been quite narrow. They often cover only crisis care, and many have no coverage for inpatient service. Some HMOs and their managed mental health care vendors have narrowly interpreted the chronic care and noncompliance exclusions for mental health and substance abuse benefits, and that has led to the frequent referral of patients to the public sector. Some outpatients have been told after three to four visits that they now have a personality disorder, are therefore chronically ill, and are not eligible for benefits. Although not all HMOs have responded in this manner, many have, and this response has given a bad name to the managed care industry in general.

Changes in the Hospital Industry

As inpatient providers have accepted the reality of managed care, they have made substantial modifications in their practice patterns. Concomitantly, the combined pressure of provider lobbying, lawsuits, improved standards, and employer demands has led to alterations in the conduct of the managed care industry. These changes are leading to increased collaboration among providers, insurance companies, and managed care practitioners. In this section, I outline some of these key trends and then conclude with some perspectives about the future.

Hospitals Have Developed Continuums of Care

Most inpatient providers have moved to develop alternatives to hospital care—often creating a continuum of treatment services including day treatment, crisis services, and group homes. Hospitals have been able to offset some of their revenue losses in the inpatient area by shifting patients into outpatient programs even though the profit margins are narrow. Many hospitals have closed units or have utilized these empty wards for alternative services. By providing a range of services, hospital providers have become more attractive to managed care companies. The managed care agencies have been reluctant to place inpatient facilities in their preferred provider networks if they have only one level of care available. Their fear is that the hospitals will be reluctant to move people into the appropriate level if they don't provide the whole range of services.

Hospital Systems Are Becoming Managed Care Companies

As hospitals have developed systems of care, they have begun to bid on or accept managed care contracts. Although some insurers and employers have been suspicious of provider- or hospital-dominated managed care services, others have welcomed this trend. Of interest is the fact that one of the larger managed mental health care companies, Preferred Health, was started by a large for-profit psychiatric hospital: Four Winds Hospital in New York. Inpatient providers who have a well-developed administrative infrastructure and a range of outpatient services are well positioned to offer cost-effective services to local employers. As the administrative demands on managed care companies increase, the hospitals that became managed care companies will need to develop the internal capacity to maintain a competitive stance.

Movement to Shorter Lengths of Stay

Most psychiatric hospitals and substance abuse facilities have substantially dropped their lengths of stay, at times by more than 50%. These trends, coupled with the diversion of some patients to outpatient programs, have led to decreased occupancy, closing of hospitals, and increased financial pressures. The reduced lengths of stay have also led to less oversight by managed care and utilization review companies as there is less need for intensive utilization review. Again, this trend has been more pronounced in the psychiatric facilities compared with some substance abuse programs.

Individualization of Treatment

Clearly, most hospitals have moved away from the nonindividualized, rigid patterns of treatment that were prevalent in the 1970s and 1980s, even though current practices vary widely from hospital to hospital and by geographic area. There has been a decrease in the practices of keeping patients for a fixed number of days for evaluation and of only arranging leaves of absence on weekends. Many substance abuse inpatient programs have moved away from the rigid 28-day model and have flexible lengths of stay tailored to the needs of individual patients. Again, these trends have decreased the degree of conflict between managed care companies and hospitals.

A More Cooperative Attitude

There has been a clear trend toward hospital providers working more co-operatively with utilization review professionals in managed care companies. The shouting matches and legal threats that accompanied the utilization review interactions with inpatient providers are significantly less frequent, even though they still occur. Disagreements over lengths of stay and intensity or appropriateness of treatment plans still occur, but the tone of the dialogue is often more civil and respectful on both sides.

Changes in the Managed Care Industry

In addition to some of the trends occurring in the hospital industry, many changes have also taken place in managed care companies.

Public Criteria

Most managed care companies have now made their medical-necessity criteria public due to legislative pressure, employer requests, and provider lobbying. This change has increased the accountability of managed care companies because they have to publicly defend and explain their decisions regarding level of care.

Increased Physician Involvement

Psychiatrists have begun to play a more integral role in many utilization review firms—especially in the larger and more respected managed mental health care and substance abuse companies. Firms such as Biodyne, which began with a model that de-emphasized psychiatrist involvement, have changed their practices over the past several years. Some companies (e.g., Green Spring Health Services) have even offered 100% psychiatrist review of inpatient care. It is relatively rare that managed care companies have nonphysicians denying inpatient care. Some managed care companies have not adopted these standards and are using physicians who are not psychiatrists to review psychiatric care. Many states have passed utilization review legislation that requires physicians to make denials and also mandates reviews by specialists.

Utilization Review Accreditation Commission

During the 1980s, utilization review and managed care constituted a relatively unregulated industry, but this situation has changed rapidly, with state after state passing utilization review bills, licensing laws, statutes regarding preferred provider organizations, and so forth. Concomitantly, the managed care industry, in association with national provider and consumer groups, has moved to create national standards and a voluntary accreditation process. The Utilization Review Accreditation Commission began evaluating and accrediting utilization review agencies in 1992, and its standards have provided a minimum floor for the practice of the larger managed care companies. The commission requires public criteria, clear appeals processes, expedited appeals, physician review, and consumer and provider accountability, as well as other standards that have improved the quality and accountability of utilization review companies.

Development of Preferred Provider Networks

The managed care industry is moving rapidly away from relying primarily on utilization review to the development of selective networks. Generally, insurance companies and employers can decrease the amount of utilization review when they use more selective, cost-effective networks. Use of these networks has reduced considerably the adversarial relationship between hospitals and managed care companies. Hospitals generally desire to join preferred provider networks in order to get referrals. They now view managed care companies as a source of revenue rather than only as a threat to revenue. Many hospitals have developed more cost-effective services and more stringent internal utilization review procedures to position themselves to be part of preferred provided organizations and other networks. To control costs, managed care companies are increasing their reliance on credentialing and privileging mechanisms, outcome studies, and provider profiling techniques, thereby reducing reliance on the inherently adversarial nature of utilization review.

The Future

Any speculations about the future of managed care companies and hospitals must consider the likelihood that President Clinton will radically revamp the health care system. Some of the health care reforms under review would drive managed care companies and hospitals into even closer collaborations. As a psychiatrist and an executive in a large managed mental health care company, I would speculate in the following manner about the future:

1. Hospitals will continue to develop networks of their own and offer a system of care. Hospitals will begin to look more and more like managed care companies as they develop the administrative infrastructure to "manage" their own patients effectively within an internal system. Hospital systems will increasingly bid for managed care business and compete with the insurance companies and managed care agencies.

2. Managed care companies will move in the direction of providing care directly or will have partnerships with hospitals and larger provider groups. Managed care companies will increasingly subcapitate with hospitals or other large provider groups, thereby reducing the need for utilization review. That will shift the role of the managed care company to one of oversight, quality assurance, measuring of outcomes, and profiling.

3. There will be significant consolidations in the managed care industry as smaller mental health and substance abuse firms are bought by larger ones and as larger medical-surgical health care companies (i.e., HMO chains) and insurance companies acquire the larger managed care mental health and substance abuse agencies. This trend has begun to accelerate in the early 1990s. Most of the larger insurance companies and HMO chains—for example, CIGNA, Aetna, and United Health Care— have acquired managed mental health and substance abuse companies and have expanded these services to all of their blocks of business. The larger companies will be differentiated to a great degree by their capacity to collect and analyze health care information and to measure outcomes and quality.

4. Higher-quality hospital systems that are cost-effective will have significant leverage in the future in their negotiations with managed care companies because they will offer significant advantages to these agencies.

In summary, it is very clear that the most difficult and contentious phase in the relationship between hospitals and managed care mental health and substance abuse companies is ending. The managed care companies that went to extremes in denying hospital care and that didn't recognize the value of inpatient services often lost business and market share and will be less competitive in the future unless their practices change. The hospitals that weren't providing cost-effective care often lost significant amounts of revenue and either have changed or have continued to lose business. As a managed care executive working in a company that has always believed that inpatient care is a critical and essential part of the continuum, I see this development as positive. If this trend continues, I can only hope that the next generation of hospital systems of care will need *less* managed care provided by outside companies.

The Clinician's View

GLEN O. GABBARD, M.D.[*]

Of all the influences on the practice of hospital psychiatry in the last few decades, none have been as sweeping and as profound as managed care. The inability to meaningfully apply diagnosis-related groupings to psychiatric disorders created a dilemma. Given the vast individual differences in patients that influence the severity, course, and treatment needs of psychiatric illness, how could regulation of cost and length of stay be performed rationally? Because of the extraordinary difficulties in finding easy solutions to this dilemma, psychiatry as a profession may have been buoyed by a false sense of security, as though psychiatric hospitals were immune to the scrutiny and control of the external review and limitation systems applied to the rest of medicine. Psychiatry was left unmanaged

---

[*]Director, C. F. Menninger Memorial Hospital, and Vice President for Adult Services, The Menninger Clinic, Topeka, Kansas; Clinical Professor of Psychiatry, University of Kansas School of Medicine, Kansas City, Kansas.

and with limited accountability. Peer review failed to limit inpatient stays because of the ambiguity inherent in measurable objectives applied to psychiatric treatment.

In this climate of nonaccountability, hospital beds for psychiatric disorders and substance abuse proliferated. In many cases, well publicized in the media, gross abuses occurred. Patients with generous insurance policies were exploited by some unscrupulous and greedy entrepreneurs who had little or no concern about the quality of treatment provided. From the perspective of the general public, the illnesses with which psychiatry deals are frightening and ill defined. Quality is difficult to measure, so third-party payers and the public placed their faith in clinicians and hospitals.

When abuses began to emerge, society began to shift its view of psychiatric hospitalization. Inpatient psychiatric treatment came to be viewed as expensive, unmanageable, and unnecessary. The problematic and complicated treatment of adolescent drug abusers became a nidus for public outrage. Considerations of cost soon superseded considerations of quality. Much of the polarization between psychiatric hospitals and managed care today has resulted from psychiatry's failure to articulate the specific dimensions of quality and outcome. Who needs treatment, and why, has also been poorly delineated. The social and occupational costs of mental illness are extraordinary, but we have done a poor job of educating public policymakers. As a result, managed care has rapidly proliferated, even in the absence of empirical evidence that it controls costs. According to some estimates, the growth of administrative costs related to managed care have now produced a situation in which one-quarter of U.S. health care spending is devoted to administration.

Impact on Staff, Patients, and Families

The impact of managed care on the staff members of the C. F. Menninger Memorial Hospital, a tertiary care referral center for treatment-refractory patients, has created a series of transformations. The initial reaction of the staff was a combination of shock and outrage at the intrusion and scrutiny of outside agencies that had no day-to-day knowledge of the patient. The anger led initially to a highly adversarial response to the challenges of the psychiatrist's professional judgment inherent in the utilization review process. A widespread feeling among psychiatrists was that their professional autonomy was no longer respected. Menninger psychiatrists have been trained to make a thorough diagnostic assessment and develop a comprehensive treatment plan based on the individual patient's needs—apart from financial considerations or the involvement of reviewers who are distant from the treatment. Many were unprepared for and resistant to the impingement of managed care.

When it became clear that managed care was not a transient nuisance that would soon go away, the outrage and shock gradually changed to demoralization at the loss of professional autonomy. In many cases, psychiatrists were being told by a utilization reviewer who was a psychiatric nurse to change their treatment plans or discharge a patient. Along with the erosion of morale, many of the clinical staff noted an erosion of the therapeutic alliance with their patients. Confidentiality between clinician and patient was no longer sacrosanct. An ambience of mistrust began to develop on the inpatient units. Patients thought that the clinical staff were no longer exclusively concerned with their progress in treatment—instead, they were increasingly concerned about complying with the demands of the managed care company reviewing the treatment.

One impact of the increasing scrutiny from outside agencies was the development of a pseudoalliance between patient and staff based on externalizing all aggression and anger onto the outside reviewer. Many of the treatment-refractory patients in the hospital carried a diagnosis of borderline personality disorder and were thus characterologically prone to engage in splitting, or dividing persons in their environment into "good objects" and "bad objects." Reviewers from managed care firms were ideally suited to become the bad objects because of their apparent lack of sympathy for the patient's need for treatment. Although directed otherwise, clinical staff were often tempted to collude with the patient in this scapegoating process because of a shared anger at the managed care company. Moreover, from the clinicians' perspective, the development of a pseudoalliance in the service of anger at a "common enemy" may have seemed far preferable to dealing with the hateful transferences of the patient.

Psychiatrists working on inpatient units reported a pervasive sense of anxiety that patients would be discharged prematurely at the behest of managed care companies only to commit suicide or otherwise decompensate. Anxiety was experienced even more intensely by the patients. One patient said she thought that she was going through treatment with "the Sword of Damocles over my head." If she didn't get better quickly, she would be "kicked out" by the managed care reviewer because she clearly could not use hospital treatment productively. On the other hand, she thought that if she showed any improvement at all, she would also be forced to leave the hospital prematurely because she would be viewed as no longer needing hospital treatment. She dreaded losing the support system of the inpatient staff and became more suicidal each time she contemplated discharge. The utilization reviewer called the patient's doctor every other day, and the feeling of being scrutinized became so intense that the patient found she could not concentrate on her treatment goals because of the constant fear that her treatment would be terminated. The psychiatrist eventually added the review process itself to the problem list in the medical record because the reviewer's scrutiny had become a major stressor for the patient and a major obstacle to the treatment process.

The anxiety of having to make profound changes in a short time is shared by both patients and staff working in inpatient settings under the watchful eye of managed care. Inpatient staff members, who are concerned that the patient may be discharged while still suicidal, often convey a "hurry up and change" attitude to the patient. These high expectations may sometimes have the paradoxical effect of making the patient decompensate. The demand to make changes that seem impossibly difficult often presents the patient with a repetition of early experiences when parents expected more of the patient than was humanly possible because of the patient's limitations.

Families of mentally ill patients have been adversely affected by the rise of managed care in a number of ways. Many have felt a sense of betrayal when the benefits they expect from their insurance policy are not available, even though all their premiums have been paid and their loved one is clearly seriously ill. Because of their feelings of frustration and impotence, families may take out their anger on employers or hospital staff. The decrease in length of stay demanded by managed care reviewers often places the burden of care on family members. Parents commonly feel overwhelmed and enraged at the prospect of caring for a mentally ill child or young adult without the requisite skills and training to know what to do. Some parents have had to quit their jobs so they could be available around the clock to take care of their disturbed family member.

Major Areas of Conflict

As the Menninger Hospital's staff realized that managed care was here to stay, they began to see that constructive collaboration was by far the best approach to working with outside reviewers. We increased educational programs for staff psychiatrists and other mental health professionals to heighten awareness of the principles of managed care. We welcomed case managers and executives from managed care firms to our campus to demonstrate our treatment programs and to openly discuss potential differences in perspective. We also have made significant changes by increasing our capacity to provide a full continuum of care. Our total number of inpatient beds decreased, whereas nonhospital and "stepdown" alternatives increased. Clinicians on inpatient units have used the appeal process when they thought that they were being pressed to discharge patients prematurely, and their point of view has been respected and accepted. Likewise, clinicians have discovered a favorable response in negotiating a reasonable continuum of care when appropriate.

Despite these areas of accommodation and collaboration, major conflicts have persisted. Perhaps the major source of tension between the hospital staff and the managed care firms revolves around the cost-versus-quality issue. Many buzzwords and phrases in the managed care lexicon, such as "managed competition," seem to be euphemisms for "cheapest available." Provisions for quality may not be taken into account. Some managed care firms define quality as achieving an acceptable outcome at the lowest possible price. An everyday problem faced by inpatient psychiatrists is that the all-inclusive, capitated rate contained in the managed care contract is not sufficient to cover the costs of treatment. A flat discounted rate is paid per day, regardless of the patient's treatment needs. If a diagnostic study, such as magnetic resonance imaging, is needed to rule out an abnormality of the brain or if around-the-clock "special" nurses are required to keep the patient from committing suicide, these additional expenses will not be reimbursed. To make matters worse, even the basic complement of inpatient staff may have to be reduced because the discounted rate is not sufficient to meet salary expenses. The treating psychiatrist is then faced with the choice of providing unreimbursed treatment or delivering lower quality care than what the situation requires.

Another significant source of conflict involves the criteria used for utilization review and medical necessity. Clinicians are concerned primarily about the accessibility and the validity of these criteria. Although some managed care companies now make their criteria available to interested clinicians, many will not reveal them. Those criteria that have been reviewed by inpatient psychiatrists are sometimes reasonable and sometimes based on a "cookbook" model that seems only peripherally related to clinical realities.

Perhaps the chief arena of conflict is one that has both philosophical and practical ramifications. The notion that psychiatric hospital treatment should be reserved for "acute medical necessity" leads to a model of hospital treatment consisting of rapid pharmacological stabilization and discharge within 7–10 days. Clinicians working in inpatient units realize that this is a largely mythical treatment model designed for a mythical psychiatric patient. In most cases, patients are hospitalized because they are not compliant with medication and other aspects of their treatment plan. The hospital unit provides the patient with an opportunity to benefit from an interpersonal holding environment not possible in outpatient settings. Psychosocial factors involved in noncompliance and decompensation can be understood and addressed in such an environment.

Psychiatric treatment simply does not lend itself to a surgical model involving a specific disease entity, a specifically tailored intervention, and a specifically predictable number of days spent in recovery. The majority of patients who are seriously disturbed enough to require hospitalization resist their treatment in a myriad of ways. To prevent repeated episodes of noncompliance and rehospitalization, the psychosocial reasons for the patient's resistance to treatment must be addressed in addition to stabilizing a self-destructive crisis. "Treatment resistant" is not synonymous with "custodial." For many patients, the safe structure of a holding environment is crucial, so that sufficient time and attention can be given to understanding the patient's reluctance to change.

Studies suggest, for example, that over half the women admitted to inpatient units have been abuse victims. The suicidal feelings of these patients are intimately related to the trauma they suffered. One 28-year-old woman thought that suicide was the only way to eradicate the horrific memories of her father's incestuous relationship with her, a daily occurrence from age 7 to age 14. She had been in and out of hospitals for brief stays with no improvement. Only when she was allowed to stay for 3 months was she able to develop a network of supportive relationships that enabled her to reexperience and work through her past trauma. She finally overcame her wish to kill herself and was able to be treated in an outpatient setting.

As long as the acute-stabilization philosophy persists, we will continue to have a revolving-door situation in which the cost of repeated brief hospitalizations will ultimately exceed the cost of one extended hospital treatment that is more comprehensive and focused. Managed care companies and mental health policymakers need to be aware that numerous problems are inherent in an acute-stabilization approach, including difficulties returning to the workplace, increased medical costs because the psychiatric problems have not been adequately treated, divorce, family disruption, and so forth.

Another aspect of this philosophical difference centers on the posthospital environment. Clearly, length of stay cannot be considered in a vacuum. Many reviewers demand that as soon as the patient is no longer acutely suicidal, transfer to a partial hospital setting must take place. An extreme example of this philosophy occurred recently in the Menninger Hospital when a reviewer told a psychiatrist, "If the patient doesn't need to be in restraints, he can be transferred to a day hospital." Although that conceptualization of the purpose of psychiatric hospitalization is in itself controversial, a more fundamental problem is that reimbursement for day hospitalization and other nonhospital alternatives is still highly variable. Psychiatrists in the Menninger Hospital and elsewhere are repeatedly faced with the dilemma that discharge is being demanded but no funding is available for less-intense forms of treatment.

Toward a Solution

Psychiatric hospitals have increasingly acknowledged that collaboration with managed care is a necessity. Unyielding polarized positions are useless and counterproductive. The time for compromise, negotiation, and collaboration is at hand. Based on our experience at the Menninger Hospital, several constructive proposals for change should be considered:

1. **Case-by-case utilization review is costly, unwieldy, unnecessary, and needlessly adversarial.** Parameters or practice guidelines (such as those the American Psychiatric Association is implementing) that take quality into account and allow for flexibility need to be established. In such guidelines, outliers must be considered, and noncustodial treatment-resistant patients must be factored in. Once such consensually established parameters are in place, then meaningful criteria for the utilization of services can be developed.

2. **Curtailing the length of inpatient stays can result in significant savings.** These savings are possible, however, only if insurance companies and the managed care firms they hire are willing to provide reimbursement for a full continuum of care. More than lip service is needed in this area. Universal standards for inpatient and partial hospital care will be helpful in making such coverage possible.

3. **Utilization review criteria must be placed on the table and made the subject of open and thoroughgoing discussion.** A dialogue between members of the psychiatric profession and representatives of the managed care industry may lead to negotiated consensus.

4. **Arbitrary demands for discharge must be replaced by reasonable collaboration.** If disagreement exists between clinician and reviewer, a site visit by the reviewer—in which a discussion with the patient, the patient's family, and the treatment staff takes place—should be standard practice. Careful assessment is needed in such situations to determine whether or not the family can adequately care for the patient after discharge. If they cannot, other alternatives need to be reviewed.

5. **If case-by-case utilization review must continue, the role of the reviewer must be redefined so that he or she becomes a member of the treatment team.** If a treatment plan could be developed through constructive collaboration between the reviewer and the staff members of the inpatient unit, then frequent review would no longer be necessary. The reviewer and psychiatrist should mutually agree on a reasonable time frame for the goals to be accomplished, and this time frame should serve as an envelope within which the treatment takes place. The patient

and family should be informed of the time parameters so that anxiety about premature termination of treatment is obviated.

6. **A mutual educational process must go on between the case management companies and the psychiatric hospitals.** Clinicians need to be educated about the crisis in health care financing so that they understand the role of managed care in preserving some health care dollars for mental illness. Managed care firms, on the other hand, need to be educated regarding the existence of treatment-refractory patients and illnesses that do not fit into standardized utilization review manuals.

7. **Finally, employers need to be brought back into the picture to better understand the disruptive effects of psychiatric illness on individuals, society, and industry.** The cost of untreated illnesses (e.g., affective disorders) should be clearly illustrated so that the decision to provide "dental rather than mental" reimbursement is no longer regarded as making good financial sense. Part of this effort to reinvolve employers should include a realistic assessment of the costs of the acute-stabilization philosophy as well.

Although outcome studies are gaining in popularity as a way of measuring the efficacy of psychiatric hospital treatment, caution is in order. Many of the approaches to outcome evaluation currently being marketed are sorely lacking in methodological rigor and are designed to be quick and inexpensive. Moreover, every clinician who has taken a fundamental research course knows that one way to improve outcomes is to treat only relatively healthy patients. The severely ill and the treatment-refractory patients may be relegated to the streets, jails, or overcrowded public hospitals in the service of improving the outcome data. I am not arguing against the implementation of methodologically sound outcome studies. I am merely pointing to the limitations of such an approach as a panacea for the current problems and tensions between managed care and psychiatric hospitals.

In the final analysis, constructive change will only come from willingness on both sides to engage in collaboration and compromise. At the Menninger Hospital, we have already experienced this rapprochement with many of the managed care firms with whom we work. The ultimate solutions will lie in mutual efforts to understand each other rather than finger pointing and blaming.

✦ 3 ✦

Intermediate Levels of Care

The Managed Care View

KENNETH A. KESSLER, M.D.[*]

The United States is engaged in a major debate over the structure of its health care system. The need to expand access to care at an affordable cost while ensuring quality will almost certainly lead to a profound restructuring of the system. In the area of mental health treatment, many innovative solutions are already in place, and others are starting to emerge. One of the changes we're likely to see is more relocating of acute-care services from hospitals to ambulatory settings. The two outpatient alternatives gaining the most attention are in-home health care and partial hospital programs (PHPs). Although there is limited experience with and less clinical literature about the former, PHPs have been successfully used to treat acute-care patients for decades, and their efficacy has been well documented. More recently, we've seen the emergence of

---

[*]Founder and President of American Psych Systems, Bethesda, Maryland; founder and former Chief Executive Officer of American PsychManagement, Rosslyn, Virginia.

freestanding PHPs that offer an alternative—rather than a supplement—to inpatient care. These developments have led managed care organizations to take a closer look at the role of PHPs in treating acutely ill psychiatric patients.

A New Role for Freestanding PHPs

The Clinical Basis

Since the early 1920s, patients with serious mental disorders have been successfully treated in PHPs. The 1963 Mental Retardation Facilities and Community Mental Health Center Construction Act mandated the role of partial hospitalization in community mental health programs. Over the next two decades, PHPs were used primarily to treat chronically ill patients in public-sector programs. During this period, the private sector's preferred treatment modality for acute-care patients was freestanding inpatient programs. To the extent that PHPs had a role in the private sector, it was principally to provide "step-down" care for patients who had received their primary treatment on inpatient units. Until recently, third-party reimbursement policies reinforced this pattern by providing more generous reimbursement for hospitalization than for alternative programs. Fearing that partial hospitalization would add to the cost of inpatient treatment rather than substitute for it, many payers did not even cover PHPs. With the advent of freestanding acute-care PHPs, this concern is being addressed.

Freestanding PHPs are likely to be the next frontier of cost savings for value-conscious payers. In addition to a record of successful experience in the public sector, the efficacy of PHPs is supported by a substantial body of clinical literature. More than 45 scientific studies have shown that PHPs produce clinical outcomes that are either superior or equal to inpatient care in the treatment of acutely disturbed psychiatric patients who do not present an imminent risk of violence. Although no study reported better outcomes for inpatient treatment, it is noteworthy that more than a third of the studies found that PHPs produced better clinical results. The authors of a major review article in the *American Journal of Psychiatry* concluded that "until . . . third-party payors economically direct patients and physicians toward partial hospitalization, the underutilization of this therapeutically and economically proven treatment modality will continue" (Parker and Knoll 1990, pp. 156–160).

The Financial Benefits

As the cost of inpatient treatment escalated in the 1980s, employers began to engage vendors with specialized skills in administering mental health benefits. In its infancy, managed care employed case management to reduce costs by decreasing inpatient length of stay. The next tool used by managed care to reduce costs was negotiating discounts with facilities and professional providers. The combined impact of case management and provider discounts dramatically lowered inpatient costs. A Foster Higgins survey reported that the average large employer spent $280 per employee per year (PEPY) for mental health benefits in 1988. Of this total, approximately $225 PEPY was for inpatient treatment. Managed care clients saw their inpatient costs reduced from $225 to approximately $85 PEPY. Savings from further reductions in length of stay or deeper facility discounts are likely to be marginal. If managed care is to impact current levels of claims expenses while preserving benefits, the savings will come from diverting hospital admissions and relocating care to ambulatory settings. I estimate that substituting acute partial hospitalization for inpatient treatment will generate an additional 33% savings over that currently realized by managed care; this reduction translates to an incremental savings of $28 PEPY. The impact of managed care on employers' inpatient mental health claims expenses is shown in Figure 3–1.

The consensus in the field is that partial hospitalization can be substituted for inpatient mental health treatment in two-thirds of the cases of hospital admission. One-third of the patients can be diverted to PHPs without first being admitted to a hospital, whereas another one-third can be treated in PHPs after being stabilized during a brief hospital stay (i.e., 1–3 days).

The Distinction Between Freestanding and
Hospital-Based PHPs

It is necessary to distinguish among different types of PHPs if the goal is to substitute partial hospitalization for inpatient treatment. The most crit-

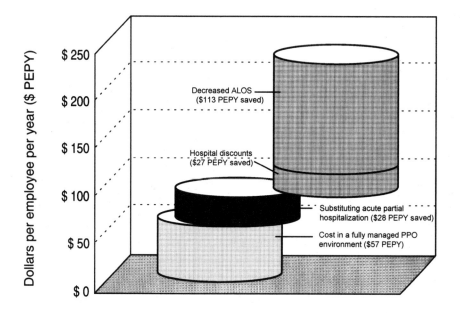

Figure 3–1. The impact of managed care on inpatient mental health expenses. ALOS = average length of stay; PEPY = per employee per year; PPO = preferred provider organization.

ical distinction is among programs that treat acute-care cases ("hospital diversion"), subacute cases ("step-down"), and chronic cases ("long term"). Although identifying long-term programs is straightforward, the distinction between hospital diversion and step-down care is, at best, ambiguous. The lack of a PHP taxonomy has created confusion about the proper role of PHPs and thereby has diminished their usefulness to managed care. Case managers have asked for guidelines about which type of patient should be referred to which type of PHP.

Until an accrediting body or the American Association for Partial Hospitalization develops operational criteria to categorize programs, the simple guideline discussed below may prove useful. This guideline addresses whether a PHP is freestanding or hospital affiliated. This is a critical distinction to make because many observers feel that freestanding PHPs offer the only real chance of systematically substituting partial hospitalization for inpatient care. The reason is simple: freestanding PHPs treat both acute and subacute cases, whereas hospital-affiliated PHPs almost exclusively treat patients after discharge from an inpatient unit. Although there are some notable exceptions among PHPs that are affiliated with a hospital, especially those associated with not-for-profit general hospitals, most provide step-down care for patients who received their primary treatment on an inpatient unit. The reasons for this exclusivity are, as my calculus professor used to say, intuitively obvious. Hospitals have major financial investments in and ongoing commitments to their inpatient services. These financial obligations do not conveniently vaporize when the need for inpatient beds decreases by as much as 50%.

A look at the recent history of some of our leading corporations may—by analogy—help to explain why hospitals are unlikely to voluntarily change their way of doing business. For more than a decade, Detroit continued producing large, poorly built automobiles with high fuel consumption despite clear evidence that the American public preferred its cars to be smaller, better built, and more fuel efficient. Detroit ignored its customers' preferences and, as a result, allowed Japanese imports to gain a large share of the American market. Another example illustrates how even our best companies have great difficulty adapting to profound changes in their markets. Many analysts believe that IBM's attachment to mainframe computers at a time when customers were shifting to microcomputers was a major cause of that company's recent problems.

The logic demonstrated by these examples is easy to see but hard to accept: mature organizations have great difficulty changing their core mission, especially when that change entails the pain associated with profound economic restructuring. Although PHPs have been shown to be more cost-effective and to produce better outcomes, hospitals are unlikely to give up their investment in bricks and mortar or to recast themselves as nimble-footed PHPs that compete with inpatient units. In general, hospitals are likely to temporize in an effort to avoid the pain and to try to preserve their investment by promoting inpatient care as the treatment of choice. It would be very surprising, therefore, if very many hospitals see their PHPs as anything more than an extender of care that supports the hospital's main business: inpatient treatment. By contrast, freestanding PHPs have no such commitment to inpatient care. Indeed, freestanding PHPs do not have a favorable long-term prognosis unless they succeed in their core mission—that of displacing hospitals as the provider of choice for the majority of acute-care patients.

In short, this is a zero-sum game: freestanding PHPs cannot grow without forcing hospitals to contract. If freestanding PHPs succeed, the market will reposition hospitals to a more limited and specialized role: they will 1) treat tertiary care cases and 2) provide brief stabilization (1–3 days) for a minority of acute-care cases before transfer to a partial hospital.

With a few exceptions, the distinction between the mission of hospital diversion and the mission of step-down care correlates reasonably well with the distinction between freestanding and hospital-affiliated PHPs. Managed care may find that determining whether a PHP is freestanding or hospital affiliated is a useful way of starting to identify programs whose mission is diverting hospital admissions. Thus, managed care will be able to identify providers that support its goals and, therefore, will be good long-term partners. With more operating experience in working with PHPs, managed care is likely to accumulate data that will enable it to assess a PHP's mission irrespective of whether the PHP is affiliated with a hospital.

Treatment in a PHP

Crisis Evaluation Service

To appropriately triage patients when they enter the health care system, some PHPs have begun to offer a crisis evaluation service. This alternative to an emergency room is the key to diverting admissions from hospitals to freestanding PHPs. If patients are to be admitted directly to a PHP, it is crucial that both they and their families see treatment in a PHP as equivalent to or better than inpatient care, not as a partial solution.

Who Can Be Treated in a PHP?

Freestanding PHPs are designed for seriously ill patients who meet criteria for hospital admission but who do not require 24-hour-a-day confinement. Acute-care patients who require intensive, multidisciplinary treatment are appropriate referrals, provided they present no immediate risk to themselves or others and have a consistent place to live. Patients in partial hospitalization programs are similar to inpatient populations, with serious mental disorders ranging from suicidal thoughts to frank psychosis. Perhaps recounting the story of a patient treated in a PHP will help to illustrate the degree of pathology that can be successfully managed without 24-hour confinement.

> The patient was referred from a staff model health maintenance organization (HMO) as a trial use of an after-school program instead of inpatient treatment. Before admission, the patient had exhibited increased symptoms of depression, was isolating himself, and was doing poorly in school. The father had raised the patient and his brother alone after the mother had abandoned them to the father's care. As the patient's behavior became increasingly oppositional, communication between the father and the patient deteriorated. The incident that precipitated admission was when the patient was severely beaten by several peers. In treatment, the patient was able to discuss feelings of sadness about being emotionally abused and abandoned by his mother. The patient also explored his poor self-image, which was reinforced by his being overweight and having a learning disability. Coping strategies were identified, the patient's behavior improved, symptoms of depression decreased, and communication with the father was reestablished. The patient and his father were both reluctant to leave the program but were helped to make the transition to outpatient therapy after the 15 treatment days originally approved by the HMO.

Differentiating PHPs From Outpatient and Inpatient Treatment

Traditional office-based outpatient treatment rarely is sufficient to meet the needs of acutely ill patients. These patients typically require intensive treatment lasting at least 6 hours daily, 5 days a week. Yet only a minority of them require hospitalization. Those that do need 24-hour confinement in addition to an intensive treatment program.

To understand the implications of separating intensity of service from a need for 24-hour confinement, it may be useful to examine how this distinction impacted the delivery of other medical services. Ten years ago, surgery was largely an inpatient procedure; today, more than 50% of surgeries are performed on an outpatient basis. This change, and the proliferation of outpatient surgicenters that accompanied it, would not have occurred without a paradigm shift; that is, the medical profession and its patients had to accept that surgical suites housed outside of hospitals were a safe alternative. In effect, once intensity of service was differentiated from 24-hour confinement, surgery no longer had to be done in a hospital. The conditions that led to a massive restructuring of surgical services in the 1980s are present in the mental health field today; the results are likely to be quite similar.

Staffing

The Joint Commission on Accreditation of Healthcare Organizations and the American Association for Partial Hospitalization recommend PHP staffing levels that are identical to those of an inpatient unit. The recommended patient to staff ratio is 4:1 for adults and 3.5:1 for adolescents. Because PHPs manage severely ill patients without a locked door, some have suggested that a higher level of clinical skill is needed in PHPs than in most hospital programs. Paul Lefkovitz, president of the American Association for Partial Hospitalization, recommends that 70%–100% of a PHP's clinicians have a master's degree (Lefkovitz 1993).

Scheduling

Fitting the program to the patient, rather than the patient to the program, is the key to a successful PHP. A flexible approach to both scheduling and programming is necessary to accommodate managed care's desire for the shortest possible length of stay compatible with a good clinical outcome. The first week of treatment in a PHP is usually the most intensive and therefore typically requires attendance 5 days a week. Starting with week 2, PHPs can begin shifting patients from 5 days a week to intermittent scheduling as the patient's condition permits.

Programming

PHPs employ the same treatment modalities as inpatient programs, including individual therapy, family counseling, occupational therapy, group therapy, and psychoeducational groups. At first glance, a day in a PHP will look much like a day on an inpatient unit. However, PHPs differ from inpatient programs in that they use a variety of strategies to minimize patient regression and dependence. One strategy is to encourage patients to stay involved in their family life and to return to routine living arrangements as early as possible. Another strategy is for treatment to be focused on a problem-solving approach in the here and now, rather than an analytic pursuit of the there and then. Yet another strategy to discourage dependence is actively transitioning patients from more-intensive to less-intensive programs within the PHP.

The core program in a PHP is the full-day program. With 6–8 hours of programming per day, 5 days a week, the day program is a suitable alternative to inpatient treatment. As patients recover, schedules are adjusted to reflect their progress by reducing the number of days scheduled per week. Patients can also move from the full day program to less-intensive levels of care within the PHP. This movement is facilitated when PHPs offer an evening program. Typically, they offer up to 4 hours of programming four evenings a week. In general, the evening program is used as a transition from more-intensive day treatment or from inpatient programs to routine outpatient therapy. However, because of its flexible scheduling and convenient after-work hours, an evening program can also provide a temporary source of additional support to prevent a hospital admission during a crisis period in outpatient therapy.

To meet the specialized needs of adolescents, many PHPs offer dedicated all-day programs. These programs typically provide 4 hours of a therapeutic school and 4 hours of intensive therapy each day. Some PHPs also offer afternoon programs for those adolescents who require intensive treatment but are able to continue attending their community school. After-school programs typically provide 4 hours of therapeutic programming 5 days a week and coordinate the treatment they provide with a school counselor.

Patient Satisfaction and Clinical Outcomes

In order to satisfy managed care clients, it is no longer acceptable to claim the high ground of quality care without quantitative data to support the claim. Cinema verité photos of struggling adolescents working out their problems under the watchful eye of an empathic therapist are not adequate proof for value-conscious buyers. Managed care purchasers insist on tangible evidence of quality. Generally acceptable measures of quality include 1) proof of program efficacy, 2) evidence of patient satisfaction, and 3) satisfactory clinical outcomes after discharge. The quality measures used to reassure clients can also be used to improve the program. American Psych Systems has found that weekly patient satisfaction surveys have led to significant program improvements. For instance, when patient surveys showed low ratings for community meetings, staff began exploring why. When it became apparent that an early starting time (8:30 A.M.) was resulting in frequent interruptions by late arrivals, the program was rescheduled to begin at 9:00 A.M.

As discussed above, managed care purchasers require evidence of treatment effectiveness. PHPs, like other providers of acute-care services, must demonstrate that patients they admit have illnesses severe enough to justify the intensity (and cost) of their programs. Further, they must demonstrate that patients improve significantly as a result of the treatment they receive. The former requirement can be met by administering psychometric tests that assess a patient's acuity on admission. The latter requirement may be met by repeating the same tests at discharge to document clinical improvement.

Because employers are asking managed care organizations for evidence of good clinical outcomes, it is likely that managed care will ask the same of its vendors. This and related developments may push managed care in the direction taken by the Ford Motor Company and other students of Japanese business practices who have chosen to work more closely with a smaller number of suppliers. To survive in this environment, PHPs will need to become value-added suppliers that anticipate managed care's needs and then try to exceed its expectations. Payers in the 1990s—be they managed care, Health Plan Purchasing Cooperatives, or a single government payer—will insist on seeing objective measures of sustained patient improvement over time. PHPs, therefore, will want to administer a set of psychometric tests before treatment, at discharge, and at some point after the conclusion of treatment.

The Treatment of Choice for Most Acute-Care Cases

It is a managed care axiom that good care is ultimately the least expensive care, yet the evidence to support this claim has not always been evident. Managed care's interest in substituting PHPs for inpatient care may be driven by an interest in controlling costs, yet the evidence suggests that this substitution will also improve clinical outcomes. Better outcomes may be related to the fact that PHPs do not provide a 24-hour hotel function and thereby do not permit patients to regress inside of a protective cocoon. In addition, freestanding PHPs design their programming and scheduling to minimize the dependence that accompanies inpatient treatment. As managed care implements the next generation of cost controls, partial hospitalization could emerge as the treatment of choice for most acute-care cases. Two decades after the heyday of community mental health centers, the lessons learned by these centers, as described at the beginning of this chapter, may be starting to enter the mainstream of the private health care system.

Recommended Reading

Hoge MA, Davidson L, Hill WL, et al: The promise of partial hospitalization: a reassessment. Hosp Community Psychiatry 43:345–354, 1992

Lefkovitz PM: Planning and implementing a short-term partial hospitalization program. Behavioral Healthcare Tomorrow 2(1):35–39, 1993

Parker S, Knoll JL: Partial hospitalization: an update. Am J Psychiatry 147:156–160, 1990

Turner VE, Hoge MA: Overnight hospitalization of acutely ill day hospital patients. International Journal of Partial Hospitalization 7(1):23–36, 1991

The Clinician's View

RICHARD D. BUDSON, M.D.[*]

Managed care has been described in the preface of this book as an industry "whose product is cost savings to those who pay for the care,"

[*]Assistant General Director, McLean Hospital, Belmont, Massachusetts; Director, Community Residential and Treatment Program, McLean Hospital, Belmont, Massachusetts; Associate Professor of Psychiatry, Harvard Medical School, Boston, Massachusetts.

introducing "cost as a crucial element in clinical decision making." If cost savings is in fact the pervading operative mode of managed care, and is perceived as such by clinicians, then the working interface between managed care and clinicians is bound to be "associated with distress and distrust." We believe that another more positive scenario is possible. In the best case, managed care is focused not on *cost* itself, but rather on the *prevention of overutilization of services*. It is this overutilization that increases cost. Defined in this manner, managed care—when done with professional expertise—can help develop more optimal care plans by requiring the provider to focus more precisely on the essential services required by a specific patient. In this way, managed care becomes a collaborator with the provider. This collaboration is in the patient's best interest both clinically and fiscally.

Clinically, overutilization fosters regressive dependence on treaters and excessively prolonged treatments. Fiscally, overutilization squanders benefits that patients—especially those with serious, chronically relapsing mental illness—need to carefully conserve for the most serious episodes of illness requiring those services over the long haul. Ideally, then, managed care works hand in hand with providers in a synergistic manner. However, in the worst-case scenario, arbitrary, unsophisticated, rigid managed care interventions—often requiring abrupt termination of services and demonstrating little appreciation of the nature of serious chronic mental illness—frustrate and irritate the clinicians providing these services. In addition, such interventions often do serious damage to patients, anger families, cause *more* utilization of services over time, and ultimately cost the payer more.

Our Institution's Capacity to Cope With Managed Care

These concepts have been developed from the experiences gained through the operation over the last several years of an extensive array of alternatives to inpatient care that are offered by our 218-bed private psychiatric hospital. These "intermediate" services include a 174-bed community residential care program providing multiple levels of care, as well as a partial hospitalization program able to serve 117 patients daily.

The first low-cost alternatives to psychiatric inpatient care in this department were, in fact, opened fully 24 years ago in 1970, with additional facilities added through the years. Thus, these facilities were largely in place before the managed care phenomenon.

If we define managed care's ultimate expectations as providing treatment in the least restrictive setting and fostering a timely flow of patients through the levels of care, we could say that the hospital's continuum of care positioned it structurally to be well prepared for the new system of managed care. Further, the institution as a whole was familiar conceptually with the treatment philosophy of moving patients rapidly into least restrictive settings. In addition, a sophisticated Utilization Review Department was in place, with nurses advocating for the movement of patients in a timely manner through the hospital system of care. Finally, the top levels of the hospital's administration in recent years have emphasized the importance of the Community Residential Care/Partial Hospitalization Department not as "a hospital stepchild," but rather as a component of the primary-care system. This combination of structural and philosophical readiness, with intrinsic support internally from utilization review and top management personnel, has permitted our institution to cope very well with the onset of managed care. In fact, we have been frustrated too often by some insurance companies who deny conversion of benefits. They, incredibly, still believe that conversion of benefits to a less costly, less restrictive setting will be an expense "add-on."

Managed Care's Impact

At the same time, it cannot be denied that managed care has had additional impact on our institution. We are taking patients who are sicker, yet we have less time to treat them than ever before. Patients also have fewer resources than ever before. The time required by clinicians to take care of patients has been increased by the necessity of communicating with managed care reviewers frequently for concurrent review. In the past, after conversion of benefits from an inpatient setting to a less-restrictive setting by an insurance company, the review would only take place when the end of the approved term approached. We believe, at the same time, that managed care may have given a broader range of clients access to our services because managed care companies understand the nature and benefits of our type of service. We aren't sure about the long-range impact on patients, and we call for longitudinal studies of patients to determine the extent to which careful selection of timely services has benefited patients over the long haul.

Areas of Stress and Conflict

There are specific areas of stress and conflict in the interface between a providing institution and the managed care company. Some of these are major issues that reflect structural deficiencies or problems. Some are minor issues that manifest themselves at the interpersonal interface between an individual clinician and a case reviewer.

One of the biggest, and perhaps more amorphous, stresses on the providing institution is the difficulty in planning new alternative services in the face of the extremely rapid change occurring within the health care economic system. There is a feeling of constant change, flux, and almost chaos as managed care companies are competing for business, deals are being made, rates are constantly being "ratcheted down." Even newer systems of care are being attempted (e.g., providers themselves becoming specialized health maintenance organizations [HMOs] by "going at risk"—accepting prospective payments per subscriber per year for a pool of people who may not necessarily become patients, and in return guaranteeing all care in that specialty needed by any subscriber during the year). In the midst of all this flux, we are very concerned that in spite of our having created a unique care system capable of treating extraordinarily sick psychotic patients at minimal cost, demands will be made that we lower the cost even more. When discounts are asked for, there seems to be a presumption that we have built in a profit margin—we have not. It feels as if a managed care company, operating for profit, assumes that we operate by the same rules. We do not. We are nonprofit.

Structural Problems

A major problem with managed care comes specifically into play when a new case of benefits conversion is considered. This problem arises from the structural separation of the responsibilities of the managed care company, which is the locus for determining and approving the treatment plan, and the responsibilities of the insurance company, which is the locus for what the benefit package is. It is our experience that neither entity wants to take responsibility for the integration of these essential elements of the overall insurance plan. That seems to us like a peculiar irresponsibility of the insurance system, which allows crucial information to be unavailable in ways that are extremely detrimental to patient care.

In practice, after a careful treatment plan is elaborated by the treatment team and agreed to by the managed care company, the managed care company will say, "We approve of this as clinically appropriate; however, it is subject to benefits eligibility." And they will go only that far. Now, unless the benefits (including the total available amount of dollars) and the insurance-covered services are immediately known to the clinician, the patient cannot be moved into the intermediate service! And when the insurance company is called, it may well have trouble determining both what services are covered and how many dollars are left!

Illustration. The utilization review manager calls the managed care company and proposes a benefit conversion to a partial hospitalization program with affiliated residence that would dramatically shorten the inpatient stay and cost 35% of the inpatient price. The managed care person says, "Gee, that sounds good, but we just got this account and we don't know what the benefits are. We'll get back to you."

Alternatively, if we have to contact the insurance company ourselves about the conversion, the dialogue might be as follows:

Illustration. The insurance representative is told about the kind of service that will cost 35% of the price of inpatient care. He or she responds, "Oh, we've heard about those. Let me find somebody who deals with this and get back to you." Two days later, the representative calls back: "We've found a policy about these kind of things. It has to be signed off by a vice president in New Jersey." Days ensue, and the patient languishes in the inpatient bed costing three times the price of the alternative. Every day in the hospital, the patient loses 2 additional days that could have been spent in a lower-cost alternative setting!

With respect to the dollars available, it is our experience that the insurance company doesn't monitor and track in real time (currently) the extent to which the benefits are expended. This lack of information totally impedes effective patient care planning.

Illustration.   We were doing a review with a case manager at a managed care company. She approved a treatment plan, stating that it was subject to "benefits eligibility." Then she found out that the patient had a $50,000 maximum and had three previous hospitalizations, and the insurance company could not determine what had been expended to date nor what was left. Days passed before the available benefits could be determined, during which no movement could be made to implement the new treatment plan; there was total paralysis in the case.

We believe that 1) managed care companies should be responsible for knowing in each case what the benefits are in both services and dollars; 2) insurance companies must keep up-to-date records of the benefits expended and have this information accessible so time is not lost; and 3) more insurance contracts should be written to cover the entire continuum of services, including partial hospitalization and residential care at different levels, in order to minimize delays.

Case Review Issues

Our experience at the level of concurrent review is quite mixed. It is clear to us that, in the best-case scenario, the managed care company reviewer can be a distinct asset to the treatment team, providing useful collegiality. The good reviewer helps us to have tighter treatment plans, with very practical, realistic, attainable goals. The weekly or biweekly meetings help focus the treatment, most usually on the patient's functioning. Instead of psychodynamics, there is often a focus on life skills. It is very helpful to our clinician when she or he perceives the reviewer as both clinically experienced and committed to quality care. The reviewer becomes a "de facto consultant" who follows the case with the clinician, "benefiting the entire treatment." Such a reviewer is experienced by our clinician as a person who "understands the potential for regression, which could lead to much more cost to the insurance company over time without proper clinical management in the present" (C. G. Masshardt, personal communication, March 1993).

At other times, some reviewers on very complicated cases have a highly personalized reaction or response to the particular patient's circumstance.

Illustration. We had a case of a very depressed widow whose husband had been a fireman who died in the line of duty. This case was reviewed by a woman 1,000 miles away whose husband coincidentally was also a fireman. It was our clinician's impression that the case could have been funded indefinitely—such was the extent of the sympathy communicated by the reviewer.

Despite the fact that the above case was ostensibly in "our favor," we yearn for reasonable, objective, rational determinations. Imagine how that same clinician feels when she has the above case simultaneously with the following one:

Illustration. In the same program as the previously described depressed widow is a man with serious, debilitating obsessive-compulsive disorder. In this case, the reviewer's position was, "Why doesn't the man just get a job and stop thinking about all that stuff!" Services were denied.

Such unreasonable reactions from reviewers can cause distress and "a sense of isolation and despair" in a conscientious clinician (C. G. Masshardt, personal communication, March 1993). Even an appeal is complicated with uncertainty about whether the treatment ultimately will be supported, leaving the patient in clinical limbo and the program at financial risk.

Another frustrating difficulty occurs when a reviewer has an established understanding of a case and a good working relationship with the responsible clinician, and a new reviewer takes over in the middle of the treatment course. Unfortunately, this change sometimes leads to unexpected, radically different treatment approaches including both extremes—with one new reviewer saying, "Why isn't this patient in the hospital?" and another saying, "Outpatient treatment alone is adequate." This example suggests that there is inadequate preparation when cases are handed off within the managed care company. We would suggest that information about a particular case, including the treatment philosophy, be carefully shared within the managed care company cadre of reviewers before a case is transferred.

Another problem we face, especially with patients who have long-term illnesses and who are very sensitive, is a lack of adequate transition time for changes in patient programs. There needs to be a period of careful planning to prevent relapse and the reemergence of symptoms such as depression and suicidality.

Illustration.   A college student residing in our high-expectation halfway house, which costs 16% of inpatient care, was doing very well. However, the staff thought that it would be a strong risk for her to return prematurely to her college dormitory. The managed care reviewer set a date that fell on the winter break, when the patient would have to move into an almost deserted dormitory. The staff vainly advocated for a 2-week extension. Within a few days of returning to the deserted dormitory, the patient became suicidal and was placed in the college infirmary, where she slept for 2 weeks. Further deterioration resulted in rehospitalization. She had to remain at the hospital for several weeks at a much greater cost than that of the proposed original plan.

That case illustrates perfectly the loss to the managed care company when its reviewers become insensitive to the clinical realities of a particular case.

A few nuisance issues, although minor, are sometimes practical matters of inconvenience. One such issue is that we have reviewers in four different time zones. A Boston-based clinician having a reviewer in either California (3-hour time difference) or Hawaii (6-hour time difference) has some logistical juggling to make appropriate calls during a shortened span of available time.

Curiously, one of our clinicians' impressions has been that California reviewers are both more familiar with and more sympathetic to our high-expectation transitional halfway house. That reminds us of the lack of a standard of care within the managed care industry.

It should also be noted that some patients whose treatment is not covered by the managed care company, and yet who are too sick to be discharged into the community, are referred to the state hospital as a last resort. Essentially, that is cost shifting, whereby the sickest patients are abandoned by the health insurance industry and the costs are shifted to the tax payers.

Future Directions

As this manuscript is in preparation, Hillary Clinton and Tipper Gore are leading the effort to change the entire delivery of health care in the United States. It is difficult to know how much opposition this effort will meet from various sectors—Congress, the insurance establishment, and organized medicine. Assuming that major changes in the psychiatric health care reimbursement system will not be federally mandated in the near future, one can speculate on various scenarios. This section of Chapter 3 contains suggestions for improving managed care. In particular, the managed care company must take responsibility for integrating the treatment plan with the available benefits, which have to be known. The quality of the reviewers should also be improved so that they are clinically experienced and aware that insensitivity to the downside of premature discharge is hazardous to all parties.

When considering what the future holds for managed care in a larger sense, one has to acknowledge that the medical establishment has a sense that it is losing its autonomy. As a result, health care institutions are making efforts to do their own managed care. For example, psychiatric institutions are contracting directly with insurance companies to "go at risk" in a capitated system and try to manage the care themselves. The ideal in this system would be for the psychiatric institutions to share the risk with the insurance companies so that neither one profits or loses exceptionally (i.e., 50% sharing of both profits and losses). If these schemes work well, then the future of managed care companies in this sector is not bright. Perhaps the managed care companies can join more collaboratively with the psychiatric institutions. Otherwise, they may be perceived to be only another layer of cost that takes away from the care of patients. Somehow, through it all, the care of patients must be our indelible focus.

CHAPTER

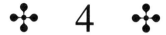

Outpatient Services

The Managed Care View

DANIEL Y. PATTERSON, M.D., M.P.H.[*]

The effort by the New York Equity Actor's Guild to cover outpatient mental health services in the 1950s serves as an interesting lesson in understanding the difficulty in providing insurance in this area. First, this effort was seminal because insurance benefits for *outpatient* mental health services were virtually unheard of until the 1960s. Second, psychoanalysis was in its heyday in the 1950s. It was in fashion for the intelligentsia to be seeing "their" analyst. As opposed to the image of psychiatrists presented in the late 1980s and early 1990s (*Dressed to Kill, Silence of the Lambs*), psychiatrists in the 1950s were depicted in the popular media as elderly, kind gurus who somehow knew the secrets and meaning of life. As you would guess, the New York Equity Actor's Guild effort was a miserable failure because of overuse: virtually every actor entered psychoanalysis for his or her "mental problems." This failed effort teaches most of the lessons as to why outpatient mental health services have been so difficult to insure.

---

[*]Private practice in psychiatry, Wilmington, North Carolina; managed care consultant.

Lesson #1. It is extremely difficult—if not impossible—to differentiate problems in living from mental illness and to differentiate efforts toward self-understanding (e.g., psychoanalysis) from the treatment of mental illness.

Lesson #2. Insuring outpatient mental health services carries a very high *moral hazard*. Moral hazard is an insurance term used to describe the vulnerability of the insurer to the insured's control over the use of the insurance benefit. The experience of the New York Equity Actor's Guild is an almost perfect example of that control. I'm sure the actors in the guild were and are still insured for cancer and other medical illnesses. Individuals do not inflict cancer on themselves or just claim to have cancer in order to use their insurance benefits.

Lesson #3. Santayana claims that those who do not know the past are doomed to repeat it. Despite the experience of the New York Equity Actor's Guild and other such experiences in the 1970s and 1980s, unions and other employee representative groups negotiated increasingly broad outpatient mental health benefits. Traditional insurers that were responsible for managing the use of these benefits were limited to only a *benefit design strategy*.

Benefit design options include the following:

1. **Benefit termination.** This was the solution of the New York Equity Actor's Guild and a solution adopted by some employers as an alternative to managed mental health care.
2. **Limitation by provider.** If the benefit says you can only see a psychiatrist and the supply of psychiatrists is limited in the geographic area where your employees live, then you can control utilization easily.
3. **Limitation by exclusion.** "Your policy does not cover marriage counseling, self-inflicted injury, etc."
4. **Visit or dollar limitation.** Your policy covers "20 visits for crisis intervention only." (See option #3.) "Your policy will pay up to $500 for outpatient mental health services."
5. **Limitation by cost sharing.** "In order to use your mental health benefits, you must meet a $500 deductible and pay 50% of visit charges."

Hard as it may be to believe, many psychiatrists and psychologists look upon these limitations and this era before managed care with nostalgia. They do so for several reasons.

First, under the indemnity insurance system, patients had free choice of providers, and mental health professionals could market themselves directly to the public and to referral sources (which they had developed over decades). Second, psychiatrists and psychologists—in a rare effort of cooperation—had been successful in keeping most of the "camp followers" (e.g., social workers, psychiatric nurses, mental health counselors) out of the insurance "tent." Third, in an indemnity system, professionals could define illness however they saw fit and could plan long-range treatment (given the limitation described above). Fourth, psychiatrists and psychologists in indemnity systems were not forced to accept assignments. Patients were usually expected to pay up front and file for benefit reimbursement themselves. Finally, mental health professionals who provided outpatient treatment covered by indemnity insurance were not subjected to quality assurance activities such as formal credentialing, chart review, and outcomes measurement. They were their own quality assurance agents, and only egregious behavior brought them to the attention of their local professional societies.

It is no wonder that these traditional mental health providers saw little they liked in managed mental health care when it hit them full force at the end of the 1980s. By then, inpatient psychiatrists and psychologists had had a good 10 years of gradual exposure to managed care. Outpatient providers began to realize that managed care was dramatically different from traditional indemnity insurance–paid care, and worse, it was acquiring a growing share of the market. Traditional outpatient providers now had to market themselves to managed care companies if they expected to get patients. These providers also began to understand that managed care companies valued camp followers such as social workers and psychiatric nurses. Therefore, psychiatrists and psychologists had to convince managed care gatekeepers that they (the psychiatrists and psychologists) had talent and capabilities that these "newcomers" didn't have. Traditional providers were asked discomforting questions about experience, training, credentials, and outcomes of treatment. Traditional providers had to give data substantiating a diagnosis and treatment plan, both by phone and in writing. Managed care companies made traditional providers sign a detailed provider contract including a fixed fee schedule that allowed no balance billing.

The days of "I'm the doctor and I alone know what is best for the patient" were over.

Managed Care Thinking

Managed care companies have struggled with and sometimes differed over the way in which to manage outpatient mental health services. It is first important to define outpatient mental health services. The frequently evoked "80/20" principle of management applies fairly well in this area. Eighty percent of patients who present for mental health care present for outpatient mental health services only. Those 80% utilize approximately 20% of the dollars allocated to mental health care. Most of those patients have diagnosable mental illness but not major mental illness. Twenty percent of patients who present for mental health care have major mental illness. Those 20% utilize 80% of the dollars allocated for mental health care.

Although more and more patients with major mental health problems will be treated in outpatient alternative settings, I will not be discussing those patients or those settings. My focus remains on the 80% who utilize only 20% of the dollars.

With outpatient services clearly defined, let me share managed care thinking about this group of patients, providers, and services—the managed care insiders' view. Before discussing management strategies, however, I want to raise issues and questions that impacted the managed care companies long before they choose a specific approach to managing outpatient services. In other words, how can managed care companies control 20% of their costs in a way that

1. **Is "quiet" for the purchasing employer.** Managed care programs that inflame local providers, generating many letters and phone calls to the company that purchased the managed care, are not looked on favorably. Managed care programs that generate employee resistance, if not outright rebellion, are also not received with favor.
2. **Minimizes the liability of both the managed care company and its client.** In the indemnity insurance world, neither the insurer nor the pur-

chasing employer is brought into medical liability suits. However, the potential for drawing a managed care company and a self-insured employer into a medical liability suit is significant. Additionally, there is the increasing problem of public relations liability (e.g., newspaper stories like "Local Widget Company employee dies of ruptured spleen after rolfing therapy sessions by company-approved therapist").
3. **Keeps outpatient providers to a manageable number.**
4. **Controls utilization.**
5. **Allows for cost-effective treatment of those outpatient mental illnesses that are treatable.**

Considerations

Managed care companies by and large employ former mental health clinicians to devise ways in which to control mental health patients and providers for the provision of cost-effective care. These clinicians understand the vulnerabilities, foibles, and gaming strategies of clinical providers. First, they understand that outpatient clinicians tend to be dedicated, well-intentioned professionals interested in the health of their patients and the public at large. However, given unlimited benefits these clinicians are endless "fine-tuners." Resolution of the problem that caused the patient to first seek care often leads to the treatment of related problems. Treatment of diagnosable illness gives way to the treatment of social, marital, or job dissatisfaction. Second, clinicians who are managed care employees recognize that even with limited benefits there is still a subtle selection for the YAWVIS patient (Young Attractive White Verbal Intelligent Successful) and away from the nonwhite, elderly, physically ill, or dying patient. Third, they recognize that there is virtually no usable outcome research that definitively favors one form of psychotherapy or one type of provider. This is in contrast to the outcome research regarding levels of care and hospital alternatives. Fourth, these managed care clinicians know how easy it is to "game" attempts to control utilization of outpatient services by insisting on a DSM-III-R non-V code[*] diagnosis or by insisting that benefits are available for couples

---

[*]V codes are used to denote conditions that are not attributable to a mental disorder but that

therapy but not for "marriage counseling." Finally, outpatient clinicians are aware that managed care companies are unlikely to review outpatient charts or to have follow-up visits with the patient to verify the information given by the outpatient provider.

Managed Care Strategies—Outpatient Care

Let me share the evolution of managed care strategies from their beginning and project what may be coming in the future—past may be prologue.

The earliest managed care vehicles were staff and group health maintenance organizations (HMOs) first developed in the late 1940s. The consumer co-op HMOs and the Kaiser Health Plans were the first to begin mental health and substance abuse programs. Initially, these programs mimicked the indemnity insurance programs in their adoption of a benefit design strategy for limiting risk, especially 1) limitation by exclusion; 2) visit or dollar limitations; and 3) in some cases, not initiating the benefit or terminating it altogether. However, to their credit, the managers of these early HMO mental health programs began to see the potential for deploying more cost-effective providers (e.g., social workers for couples counseling) and for developing and using more cost-effective outpatient alternatives to inpatient care (e.g., structured outpatient substance abuse programs).

The 1970s and 1980s saw the development of the independent practice association–health maintenance organizations (IPA-HMOs), preferred provider organizations (PPOs), and utilization review programs. These second-generation managed care organizations had (and have) the following elements in common.

Utilization Review

At its core and at its best, utilization review is based on the following steps:

---

may be the focus of attention or treatment (e.g., uncomplicated bereavement).

1. Independent and scientific determination of the efficacy of a procedure (e.g., the procedure consistently results in a desired outcome).
2. Independent and scientific determination of the appropriate indicators for such a procedure. For example, virtually all practitioners would agree that appendectomy is an efficacious procedure for the treatment of appendicitis. There are probably still arguments as to when this procedure is indicated, given the fact that rupture of the appendix can be life threatening and surely should not be the only indication for appendectomy.
3. The independently determined indicators (given that the procedure has been proven to result in a desired outcome) must be reduced to no more than a 15-minute question-and-answer telephonic review or written questionnaire.
4. If the clinician has not provided information that would justify the need for the requested procedure, the utilization review clinician must respectfully decline approval of payment for the procedure.

Selected Providers

Insurers that essentially offer indemnity insurance and that have utilization review programs often rely on a time-honored method of provider selection: limitation by provider type (see benefit design option #2, above). If you only pay M.D.'s (i.e., psychiatrists) or M.D.'s and Ph.D.'s and only review the care they render, you have combined utilization review with provider selection to reduce cost and provide more *cost-effective* care.

PPOs undertake utilization review as described in the "Utilization Review" section, but they make an effort to select "preferred providers." Rarely are such preferred providers initially chosen by the patients who are to use them. The managed care company exercises the preference for both good and questionable reasons. On the positive side, they can choose providers with the appropriate credentials for the care they render. They can also choose providers that agree with a common mission—the provision of cost-effective care. On the negative side, if the PPO only chooses providers 1) who have just the basic credentials, 2) who accept reduced fees because they can't compete in the marketplace (i.e., they have no following of patients or referral sources), and 3) who will obediently follow the directions of the managed care company even when such directions seem inconsistent with what is required to provide good care, then these PPOs are only cost-cutting organizations that are neglecting the second half of their mission—providing *cost-effective* care.

IPA-HMOs may develop their panels and review programs in the same manner and may indeed look for all the world like PPOs except for one characteristic. PPOs, if they are worthy of their name, provide an option for the patient-member to seek care outside of the preferred provider panel. IPA-HMOs do not provide this option. Ideally, the PPO creates an environment in which members will get better care for a more reasonable price (lower deductibles and copayments) than they would if they went outside the preferred provider panel.

Although provider selection operates in the mental health world as it does in the medical-surgical world, the processes of utilization review are significantly different. Even criteria for selecting a level of care and for determining differences in outcome for each level of care are hard to develop given the relative dearth of scientific information on indications and outcomes. More difficult is the task of defining usable criteria for determining when and how much outpatient treatment is needed. That difficulty notwithstanding, there is pitifully little outcome research on the effectiveness of psychotherapy. The only area that approaches the same level of sophistication as medical-surgical review is the review of indications for the use of psychotropic medications. To remove the emperor's clothes, *no utilization review program has workable criteria for reviewing outpatient care.* Even attempts to hold clinicians to the DSM-III-R criteria for diagnosis have been difficult because there is virtually no attempt to independently corroborate clinician-given diagnoses.

The most thankless, difficult job in the mental health utilization review company is the review of standard outpatient care. Although some utilization review companies use Global Assessment of Functioning scores or other similar measures for guiding utilization review efforts, most companies regress to the following common denominator. Does the clinician who is calling (telephonic review) or writing (outpatient treatment reports) sound as if he or she understands what is going on with the patient and knows what to do? Does the call or report make internal sense (e.g., does the history and mental status report substantiate the diagnosis, and does the proposed treatment fit the diagnosis)? Is the clinician realistic in his or her request for treatment sessions?

Most outpatient utilization review devolves to a form of rationing. "You want 25 sessions; let's start with 5 and review at the end of those sessions."

Toward the end of 1980, some managed care companies began to interpose an evaluator who was either an employee of the utilization review company or "bonded" to the utilization review company to serve as a face-to-face evaluator (and at times a short-term treater). The evaluator's tasks were 1) to determine that patients requesting mental health care had a diagnosis or problem meriting treatment and 2) to provide the utilization review company with a knowledgeable opinion for guiding review decisions about long-term treatment.

The Future

As I noted previously, past may be prologue. The Clinton administration has early committed itself to "managed competition" in which organized systems of care will ideally compete to offer better health care at a more reasonable price to collections of buyers organized into "purchasing cooperatives," with government providing the buying funds (premiums) for indigent and medically indigent persons. Thus, the current fee-for-service free market will be converted to an oligopsony of buyers (purchasing cooperatives) bargaining with an oligopoly of providers (accountable provider systems).

What is fundamental and inescapable about these transformations is that all practitioners operating in such provider systems will be accountable both fiscally and clinically, as well as being accountable for obtaining patient acceptance of their treatment practices. In the mental health care arena, the employees of an HMO mental health department, a group practice, a "group practice without walls," or a mental health managed care company contracting with an accountable provider system all will be dealing with the same bottom line.

That group must provide a defined set of benefits and services to a defined or enrolled population, using a fixed budget over a set period of time. As we all know, crisis is a time of danger and a time of opportunity.

The danger is that mental health and substance abuse will again get short shrift when folded back into medical-surgical organizations. The danger is that the basic set of benefits and services required by law will be modeled on the HMO Act of 1973. The danger is that broader mental health benefits will become prohibitively expensive due to changes in the tax code.

The opportunity is that all U.S. citizens will have access to mental health and substance abuse care. There is the possibility, if not the probability, that mental health care will be managed more at the local level and that the problem of delivering cost-effective outpatient service will be approached logically by those empowered to seek a solution.

The Clinician's View

ROBERT K. SCHRETER, M.D.[*]

There is emerging consensus among managers and clinicians in favor of outpatient care. This section of Chapter 4 examines the impact of managed care on outpatient services, with special attention to the challenges confronted by patients, providers, and the delivery system.

Patients

A crucial issue for clinicians and reviewers is the ability to provide outpatient services to severely and persistently mentally ill patients. Their impairment and fragility place them at risk for decompensation, requiring hospitalization. For these patients, outpatient sessions are seen as a trade-off for more costly inpatient days. There also appears to be emerg-

[*]Private practice in psychiatry, Baltimore, Maryland; Medical Director, Psych Services, Baltimore, Maryland; Assistant Professor of Psychiatry, Johns Hopkins Medical School, Baltimore, Maryland.

ing agreement that treatment of the so-called "worried well" will not be reimbursed by medical insurance.

The group of patients who are least well served by current managed care approaches are those whose illnesses are not so severe as to require hospital admission but do cause significant distress and dysfunction. On one end of this spectrum are patients with an Axis I diagnosis indicating major mental illness superimposed on Axis II pathology in the areas of developmental disability and personality disorder. On the other end of the spectrum are patients with character problems. Two case summaries are presented in order to highlight the types of patients frequently perceived by providers as requiring more intervention than managed care will allow.

Mrs. A., a 49-year-old mother of two, is referred before discharge from her fifth hospitalization in a 7-month period. Her past history was marked by erratic behavior in social, vocational, and family spheres. She complains of memory lapses and periods of blankness. During her third admission, her fragmentation showed itself to be an aspect of multiple personality disorder, with up to 18 alters identified by patient and clinicians. A contentious, demanding woman, she created chaos wherever she went. Efforts at treatment were complicated by her "doctor shopping" to locate a rescuer, her rapid disappointment in clinicians who inevitably failed to satisfy her needs, and her capacity to pit clinicians against one another.

Mrs. A. is a pervasively disturbed woman with Axis I pathology superimposed on an Axis II disorder. Her admissions become necessary when her multiple personality disorder becomes so flagrant that she cannot be contained in the outpatient setting. Like most patients, she is discharged from the hospital quicker and sicker. However, it is her underlying borderline personality disorder that makes creation of an adequate outpatient program so difficult. Similar difficulties arise in the treatment of other patients. Bipolar disorder deteriorates into mania. People become suicidal as part of a major depression. Schizophrenic patients develop acute psychosis.

Under managed care, treatment of such patients is often complicated by limiting coverage to resolution of acute episodes or by authorizing as few as four to six sessions of outpatient care at a time. Clinicians then have two options: 1) terminating care before it seems clinically sound, or 2) devoting time to filling out forms or playing telephone tag with reviewers. More generous managed care companies will authorize 10–20 sessions at a time. This practice should be encouraged when clinically appropriate. Just four to six sessions is unrealistic for some patients with diagnosable psychiatric disorder.

Furthermore, clinicians must have some flexibility to design adequate treatment programs. Patients like Mrs. A. need a three-pronged treatment approach: 1) emergency intervention for hospital diversion; 2) crisis intervention to stabilize the patient; and 3) longer-term work, often involving family, support groups, and outside agencies. This crucial longer-term follow-up is often denied by cost reviewers. Patients are left without the help they need in dealing with the stresses that often precipitate decompensation.

Mrs. B. was a 39-year-old, well-respected health professional, mother of a 9-year-old boy referred for evaluation by his school. The child was described as oppositional, combative with peers and teachers, and difficult to teach. Early in the treatment of the child, his mother came to recognize that his problems were a "ghost from her nursery." Her history revealed abandonment by her biological father before her birth and a childhood dominated by severe physical abuse as well as severe maternal rejection. Her smiling, compliant demeanor and exemplary job performance covered a seething rage that colored her every experience. She was often suicidal and had made suicide attempts at several points in her life. As his mother revealed her distress, the child seemed to settle down and she became the identified patient.

Mrs. B. presents a very different managed care dilemma. She functions at a high level in the workplace and would not be seen as having a mental disorder based on superficial evaluation of her social relationships or activities of daily living. However, the depth of her rage and depression, the intensity of her suicidal urges, and the hardships she inflicted on her family could hardly be described as "worried but well." Her disorder is neither acute nor readily encapsulated in a short-term focus. It is the result of long-term trauma that adversely affected multiple aspects of her development.

We can anticipate that a managed care reviewer would correctly recognize Mrs. B.'s difficulties as chronic and likely to require long-term treatment. Corporate culture and attention to the bottom line would encourage this reviewer to limit treatment to a short-term intervention and disregard the chronic issues. This approach would be quite inadequate for this patient's needs.

These cases highlight a number of other issues that demand attention as managed care unfolds. The so-called worried well are being denied all reimbursement for outpatient services. Their difficulties are being labeled "problems of living." Their care is increasingly seen as a social intervention rather than a medical treatment. Redefinition will not make these problems disappear. We will, therefore, need to enhance our ability to distinguish between problems of living and diagnosable medical conditions. We will also need to decide where these people will receive attention. Evidence points to a delivery system that will be demedicalized, deprofessionalized, and feminized. It is also likely that medical insurance will cease to be the primary financing mechanism for these interventions.

Another important issue is the arbitrary denial of coverage for outpatient services and the dilemma it poses for patients and providers. Entire diagnostic categories, such as attention-deficit hyperactivity disorder, are excluded from coverage. Therapeutic interventions, such as intensive psychotherapy and psychoanalysis, are often excluded from reimbursement. Outpatient sessions are limited to as few as 10 sessions per year, regardless of the nature of the disorder. Denial occurs without adequate research evidence to support these limitations. Significantly, the entire process has occurred without public scrutiny or debate.

This dilemma arises, in part, out of the manner in which managed care is marketed as a product. The patient is promised the highest quality care. The purchaser of care, whether a private employer or the government, is promised cost savings. Common sense demands recognition that these goals can be mutually exclusive. It is incumbent on the managed care industry to acknowledge this reality. Public acknowledgment of the efforts to provide the highest quality care within very real resource limitations is likely to foster open discussion among the various constituencies affected by the decisions.

This discussion must be based on the recognition that we are developing a two-class mental health system, particularly with respect to outpatient services. People of means will always be able to finance treatment out of pocket. The less fortunate will rely on the generosity of employer-financed managed services or receive care in the public sector. These people will find access to care blocked by unaffordable copayments, arbitrary limits to numbers of sessions or total dollars available in a calendar year, or other rationing mechanisms.

Providers

Outpatient psychological services have traditionally been organized around the biopsychosocial model. In this model, clinical data are synthesized from multiple areas of the patient's life. Treatment plans aim for comprehensiveness and complexity without regard to cost. Clinicians trained according to this model are under pressure to abandon it in favor of treatment based on efficiency. Efficiency can be translated as clinical care that takes into account cost-effectiveness and the bottom line. Managed care efforts at effecting this shift initially relied on utilization review to deny treatment and create a sentinel effect. Cost savings too often resulted from intimidation and exhaustion. This led to understandable conflict and animosity. A positive change has been the recent willingness of some companies to authorize treatment in blocks of 10–20 sessions. These companies reserve review and case management for the small number of cases and providers who consume the majority of the care and dollars.

Managed care executives have the advantage of a clearly defined goal. Their job is to save money for the purchaser of care, thus increasing profits for the purchaser and the managed care company. Quality of care is a means to this end for some companies.

Clinicians have a more difficult time identifying a single goal because their role is an amalgamation of often conflicting responsibilities. They are obligated both to consider their patients' well-being and to operate within the legal system that sets the standard for care (often in conflict with cost-effectiveness); they also want to generate adequate income from their practice. The Hippocratic Oath focuses on physicians' responsibility to each individual patient, in contrast to the managed care goal of shepherding resources.

Another source of conflict is the different sense of time that providers and managers bring to their tasks. Clinicians think in terms of the course of an illness, which, although it may appear in episodes, often extends over the life of the patient. Managed care contracts go from year to year. Managed care executives often think in terms of quarterly reports and yearly bonuses. At this point in our understanding of illness and management, there is no evidence to suggest that what is cheapest in the short term maintains its advantage in the long term for many disorders.

Treatment

Recently, some managed care companies have published criteria for inpatient care and the associated interpretative guidelines. These criteria lend clarity to the process—which is to be applauded. Companies that have not yet articulated their criteria should be expected to do so. There should be a similar open discussion of outpatient services and covered conditions.

Clinicians need to understand that simply doing what they have always done will serve neither patient nor clinician. The challenge for clinicians is to create innovative treatment approaches that adequately deal with patients' problems and promote change.

Therapeutic interventions in the era of managed care will increasingly be identified by the following characteristics:

❖ **Short term.** Open-ended treatment occurring weekly over a large portion of the calendar year is actively being discouraged. Crisis interventions of 5 sessions or less and brief treatments of 10 sessions are becoming the favored modality. Treatments of 10–20 sessions are now seen as longer-term interventions.

❖ **Focused.** Patients and clinicians are asked to identify a treatment focus, usually some aspect of the chief complaint. These foci can often be identified as target symptoms.

❖ **Goal oriented.** Therapeutic steps are aimed at these target symptoms. Adequate resolution of the chief complaint is seen as indicating readiness for termination. Treatment of chronic difficulties and underlying character issues is seen as beyond the scope of reimbursable psychological interventions.

✣ **Prescriptive.** Clinicians are asked to design treatment that is specific for the chief complaint. They are discouraged from simply modifying their preferred technique without regard to the presenting problem.

✣ **Episodes of care.** In the emerging model, psychotherapy is seen as a process occurring in pieces over time. Patients are asked to terminate treatment when there has been resolution of the acute problem. If this issue reemerges or additional problems develop, the patient can return for additional short-term treatments.

✣ **Outcome focused on dysfunction.** Although clinicians maintain that distress and dysfunction cannot be measured exclusively in dollars, managed care concentrates on impairment in activities of daily living.

✣ **Outcome focused on stabilization.** The goal of short-term interventions under managed care is the stabilization and return to premorbid levels of functioning and not the resolution of character issues or long-term growth.

Clinical experience suggests that short-term interventions are inadequate for as many as 20%–30% of all patients. Some have chronic or relapsing disorders that will respond to treatment over time. Others fail to improve with short- or long-term treatment. Often these refractory patients have a characterological disorder and are unwilling to accept responsibility for treatment or unable to sustain a therapeutic relationship. These "difficult patients" consume a disproportionate amount of provider time and system resources. These are the patients for whom there is the greatest temptation to manage dollars rather than care.

Clinicians and managers face the challenge of more accurately matching patient needs with treatment modalities. Innovative treatment approaches will help achieve this goal. Clinicians also must address the distinction between treatable and untreatable character disorders. In an era of cost containment, drawing this distinction will inevitably affect treatment decisions. This consequence raises troubling ethical issues that have not yet been addressed.

Survival for the Clinician

Clinicians currently in practice were trained in the era of the solo practitioner. That era has passed, probably forever. Many believe that the multispecialty mental health group is likely to become a survival mechanism for clinicians in the 1990s.

Giant corporations and government now contract with other giant corporations to provide health and mental health services through carve outs and preferred provider networks. Patients are losing the right to choose their own providers. Providers find themselves excluded from access to large numbers of patients. The individual clinician, acting alone, is poorly positioned to respond to these far-reaching changes.

By uniting to form groups, clinicians will be better able to remain players in the emerging system. These groups can be loosely organized as independent practitioner organizations or formally structured as partnerships or corporations. They can operate locally, regionally, or nationally. The public sector can participate on an equal footing through its community mental health centers. Regardless of the arrangement, these organizations must be in the position to provide services to large numbers of patients over wide geographic areas and bid directly for contracts. We must prepare for the next step in the evolution of managed care: Managed care companies will become middlemen who contract with alliances and employers. Responsibility for the actual care of patients will be parceled out to local and regional provider groups that will pay the managed care company for access to these patients and for the administrative services necessary to support their treatment.

Participation in multispecialty mental health groups offers clinicians the following advantages:

❖ The opportunity to gain access to large patient populations as a defense against exclusion from networks and carve outs.
❖ The assurance of a sizable-enough population of patients to justify the overhead associated with providing the wide range of services necessary while benefiting from economies of scale.
❖ The availability of office support services that have become necessary in current practice but that are often too expensive for solo practitioners.
❖ Utilization review that can be built into the system, eliminating the cumbersome process of dealing with external reviewers who serve as watchdogs.
❖ The ability to ensure that patient care is clinically managed rather than

fiscally managed and to ensure that the clinical perspective maintains precedence.

✥ At least some protection against the continued erosion of autonomy and control we are currently experiencing.

✥ The ability to make peer clinical and emotional support available to providers as part of the delivery system.

Conclusion

Outpatient treatments are human relationships entered into with the hope of promoting growth and change. We must use these relationships wisely. The relentless pressure to do more with less will persist. Clinicians are challenged to develop innovative treatments and to redesign the delivery system. Managers must resist the temptation to manage dollars and not care.

Recommended Reading

Budman S, Gurman A: Theory and Practice of Brief Therapy. New York, Guilford, 1988

Feldman J, Fitzpatrick R: Managed Mental Health Care. Washington, DC, American Psychiatric Press, 1992

Goodman M, Brown J, Deitz P: Managing Managed Care. Washington, DC, American Psychiatric Press, 1992

Child and Adolescent Services

The Managed Care View

RONALD GERATY, M.D.[*]

A 15-year-old youth was admitted at 3:00 A.M. on a Saturday over a holiday weekend. He had been at an all-night party after drinking heavily. His father was called by concerned friends who found the young man passed out. Finding his son intoxicated, the father believed his son had made a suicide attempt and called an ambulance. When the son was roused by the ambulance attendants to be taken to the hospital, he threatened to kill his father.

On evaluation in the emergency room, the son, his father, and his mother were all seen by the child and adolescent psychiatrist on call. Each had a slightly different perspective. The young man complained that his parents, especially his father, were overly controlling and restrictive in their rules. When he had asked to go to the party, his father refused permission, but the son went anyway. He did drink too much but took nothing other than alco-

[*]Executive Vice President of Medco Behavioral Care Corporation, Burlington, Massachusetts; Instructor in Psychiatry, Department of Psychiatry, Harvard Medical School at the Cambridge Hospital, Cambridge, Massachusetts.

hol (though drugs were available), and when he got too drunk, he fell asleep "to sleep it off." His friends got worried that he had mixed drugs and alcohol and called his dad for help. He believed his father alleged suicide as a way to get him in trouble and as a punishment. Though he admitted sometimes he would rather be dead than alive at home, he did not want to die. The threat to kill his dad had been made before, and he had even gone to the gun cabinet at home to be sure that the guns and ammunition were available.

The mother discussed her fear of the violence of both her husband and her son. Her son had been arrested for repeated fights and was on probation for "disorderly conduct." He had been seen several times at an outpatient clinic run by a managed care company. The mother did not know what the outcome of the treatment had been. She attended one family meeting, but the father had refused to go. She took her son to the clinic at the suggestion of the probation officer. The father, a U.S. Marine, had a history of violent outbursts in which he threatened her and her son. She did not know whom to fear more. Although she did not think her son was suicidal, she begged the hospital to keep him so he would not "blow up" at home. The father did not want to discuss the past but demanded that his son "be fixed" and felt that the clinic treatment had been ineffective, as he had predicted.

The patient was admitted, partially intoxicated with alcohol (by history and according to a drug screen), and admitted his anger and wish to kill his dad. He described a history of alcohol use to intoxication only twice before and no regular use. He had no other pertinent findings on physical examination, past psychiatric history, personal history, or mental status. He was admitted with a 2-day approval from the managed care company for care in the hospital. Because the emergency case manager did not have access to the clinic's records (the case manager took the call from another city), he could not verify the clinic visits or history.

On Tuesday, after the holiday weekend, the treating psychiatrist requested an extension of the hospitalization for further evaluation with family involvement, psychological testing, a trial pass to go home, a discharge treatment plan to include outpatient treatment, and a commitment not to kill his dad (the patient refused to contract not to kill his dad, although he doubted he would). The managed care company denied the request for extension of the stay, saying that psychiatric hospitalization was not necessary because the acute situation had passed and because review of the outpatient record revealed noncompliance with treatment recommendations and a history of violent outbursts that were self-limiting. The recommendation was made that the evaluation could continue on an outpatient basis. The psychiatrist appealed the decision, requested that a child and adolescent psychiatrist be the reviewer because of the developmental issues involved, and kept the patient in the hospital.

The perspective of the hospital and the psychiatrist is easily understood. The patient had been admitted on an emergency basis after an acute episode. The psychiatrist, who did not know the patient, believed that he could be suicidal or violent or both based on a middle-of-the-night evaluation and admitted him for evaluation and containment. Now, on Tuesday, the first workday after the holiday weekend, the patient needed to be evaluated completely. The hospital staff and the psychiatrist felt taken advantage of by the managed care company, which was available by telephone only during the emergency on the holiday weekend and now wanted the patient out of the hospital. Although the emergent crisis did appear to be past, the risk of another crisis could not be determined without more time. And although the case might appear more "normal" if the son were 18 rather than 15, there was significant concern that the son's behaviors were age inappropriate.

The perspective of the managed care company can also be understood. The patient had an acute episode of intoxication with belligerence that had resolved. The brief stay at the hospital had provided a safe "holding environment" away from the tensions at home. The patient's history showed similar episodes in the past (although none had required hospitalization), and, though the patient had missed several outpatient sessions over the past months, he had an outpatient therapist who was willing to treat him. Although the "severity of the illness" had warranted the admission, the "intensity of the services" over the weekend had not met criteria for an active treatment program. Now the severity of illness no longer warranted the intensity of the services offered, and the result was a denial of authorization for payment for further inpatient services.

If each perspective is understandable, what's wrong? Or rather, what solutions can be introduced so that perspectives can be joined?

The first solution has already been implied. We need more active dialogue between the parties (such as the dialogue in this book) so that we can achieve agreement about our long-term goals, which will lead to more agreement regarding our short-term differences of opinion. For example, in the previously described clinical case, both the managed care company and the psychiatrist would agree that the safety of the patient and a positive clinical outcome over time are shared goals. Both agreed that the crisis warranted hospitalization even if all criteria for admission might not have been met. The disagreement came over when to discharge the patient. Perhaps, if the outpatient therapist had contacted the hospital on Tuesday morning, shared her knowledge of the history, and offered to see the patient quickly, the treating psychiatrist might have agreed. So the first solution is to increase the dialogue among managed care companies, providers, and others to identify mutual goals even if the methods and approaches are different.

The second solution is implied as a result of the first solution. Understanding comes more easily in the context of a relationship. If the hospital and the managed care company had worked together over time and with several cases, each might have been able to understand the other's perspective more readily. If the managed care company had confidence that the clinical judgment of the hospital psychiatrist was not influenced by the wish to generate inpatient revenues with a long hospital stay or by the fear of a malpractice suit, an extension of a stay would be more likely. It is probable, however, that managed care case managers begin conversations with unknown providers with the assumption that hospitals want to keep patients, whereas hospitals assume that case managers *don't* want patients to stay. As long as conversations begin with such assumptions, it's not surprising that more extreme positions get presented.

It is for that reason that most specialty managed care companies are shifting away from "stand-alone" telephonic utilization review, whereby patients select any provider and that provider is subject to review. That approach to managing care, though prevalent today, is becoming less common. Rather, the fastest-growing approach to managing care is the preferred provider organization, in which selected providers agree in advance to work together on the basis of published criteria, shared values, and discounted fees.

The third solution is, whenever possible, to use case managers with training and experience similar to that of the provider. When the previously described case is examined from a developmental viewpoint, the patient's behavior may be seen as age inappropriate. If the managed care reviewer had been trained in child and adolescent psychiatry, the dialogue about symptomatology, diagnosis, and treatment planning in light of the developmental stage of the patient might have given the treating psychiatrist more comfort and resulted in an agreement without leading to appeal. Less than 10 years ago, most utilization reviewers were not even trained in psychiatry, let alone trained in a subspecialty. This lack of sensitivity and expertise led to the development of the managed mental health industry. The logical conclusion is that managed care companies that continue to develop case manager expertise in subspecialty areas (e.g., chemical dependency, child and adolescent psychiatry, and psychopharmacology) will be more successful both in communicating with providers and in making good decisions that result in cost-efficient treatment.

Lastly, another solution that would have helped resolve the problems presented in this clinical case would have been the existence of a full continuum of care. For instance, if an emergency foster care placement had been suggested after the initial hospitalization or if a home-care program had been available (where a child care worker could spend time in the home on a temporary basis to assist in the teenager's reintegration into the home), both the psychiatrist and the managed care company could have been more reassured that a safe environment would be possible. And if a partial hospital or intensive outpatient program had been available to take responsibility for the patient, everyone would have been comfortable with an earlier discharge.

Beyond the continuum of care (which almost everyone agrees is a good idea, whether they are in the managed care industry or in the provider industry), continuity of care is a concept that needs to be explored further. The attending psychiatrist was reluctant to discharge the patient to an outpatient therapist whom she did not know; however, if the patient could have entered a system that would manage him throughout the continuum, either through a single "attending" clinician or through contractual and functional agreements, everyone would have felt more comfortable.

This case raises a more philosophical question that has huge implications for child and adolescent psychiatric practice. Although few would believe this young man suffers from a major depression, most would agree that his symptoms fit into a general classification of aggressive or disruptive disorders (although he probably does not meet the strict criteria for conduct disorder). Aggressive behavior brings over half of all young people to treatment (O'Donnell 1985). Although the American Academy of Child and Adolescent Psychiatry's practice parameters (Jaffe et al. 1992) indicate that treatment at a psychiatric facility is appropriate for patients with conduct disorder, it lists significant risk of death or significant injury *and* failure of treatment at a less intensive level of care as criteria to be met for hospitalization. Some (Marohn 1992) advocate for psychiatric facility treatment of aggressive youths; however, newer treatment approaches build on the assumptions that the best treatment 1) occurs in the natural setting of the child's family, 2) is possible in the home, and 3) must be organized to respond to the ever-changing needs of the patients (England and Cole 1992). In the few clinical outcome studies done on such disorders, it has not been shown that psychiatric hospitalization or even traditional psychiatric outpatient treatment plays a definitive role in a good prognosis. If expensive treatment cannot be shown to produce better results than other types of incarceration, at what point should the decision be made to continue or discontinue that treatment? Of course, no one would question the need for containment to ensure a patient's or family's safety in an emergency.

One other comment must be made about this case. It is important to remember that although the child and adolescent psychiatrist may not have worked closely with the managed care company and therefore did not arrive at a treatment plan that was consistent with the wishes of the managed care company, she made the correct decision when her treatment plan was rejected by the case manager—she continued the hospitalization and appealed the decision. It's crucial that clinicians remember that they do not yield their clinical judgment even if case managers do not authorize reimbursement (Geraty et al. 1992).

Nowhere has the impact of managed care principles been more dramatic than in the area of inpatient child and adolescent psychiatry. The role of brief inpatient treatment (less than 2 weeks) has been debated

(Sarles and Alessi 1993). Although the growth of child and adolescent treatment facilities within psychiatric hospitals and residential treatment centers was dramatic in the 1980s, their reported collapse has been just as dramatic in the 1990s. However, the need for effective and efficient treatment continues unabated in the outpatient area.

The future needs of child and adolescent psychiatry lie in the area of studying clinical outcomes and comparing various clinical approaches. Recently, the American Academy of Child and Adolescent Psychiatry formed an "Outcomes and Treatment Efficacy Project" to respond to this need. This project, under the leadership of Dr. William Ayres, president of the academy, is designed to give careful study to this area and to publicize the research being done. It accompanies the development of further practice parameter guidelines such as the one referenced on conduct disorders. We owe it to our profession and to our patients to participate in this ongoing debate and dialogue.

References

England MJ, Cole RF: Building systems of care for youth with serious mental illness. Hosp Community Psychiatry 43:630–633, 1992

Geraty RD, Hendren RL, Flaa CJ: Ethical perspectives on managed care as it relates to child and adolescent psychiatry. J Am Acad Child Adolesc Psychiatry 31(3):398–402, 1992

Jaffe S, Ayres W, Bryant E, et al: Practice parameters for the assessment and treatment of conduct disorders. J Am Acad Child Adolesc Psychiatry 31(2):iv–vii, 1992

Marohn RC: Management of the assaultive adolescent. Hosp Community Psychiatry 43:622–624, 1992

O'Donnell DJ: Conduct disorders, in Diagnosis and Psychopharmacology of Childhood and Adolescence. Edited by Weiner JM. New York, Wiley, 1985, pp 249–287

Sarles R, Alessi N: Resolved: two-week hospitalizations of children are useless (debate forum). J Am Acad Child Adolesc Psychiatry 32:215–220

The Clinician's View

ALAN A. AXELSON, M.D.[*]

Child and adolescent mental health services have always been shaped by external forces. Trends in the 1970s expanded children's entitlements to special education and psychiatric services. This expansion, coupled with an increase in the availability of insurance for inpatient services, resulted in increasing utilization of inpatient treatment services in the 1980s. The highly visible dollars flowing to psychiatric units in general hospitals and freestanding facilities—and the variability in the criteria for treatment—spawned a major business opportunity in behavioral managed care. In its simplest form, preadmission and concurrent review via telephone determines on a case-by-case basis whether or not payment will be authorized for particular services.

The authorization for inpatient services is based on meeting criteria that are generally related to dangerousness and are very similar for children and adults. The results have been dramatic, with major reductions in child and adolescent inpatient services and a major restructuring of services. The application of the criteria—if not the criteria themselves—varies from one managed care company to another. With some companies, the objective is dramatically restricting the utilization of inpatient services. Other organizations are more focused on developing effective, cost-efficient treatment for a particular patient. The complexity of working with a number of different companies with varying criteria and procedures contributes to the cost and administrative frustration associated with delivering clinical services. The common denominator is that the providers of service work harder for lower fees.

[*]Medical Director and Chief Executive Officer, InterCare–Comprehensive Behavioral Healthcare, Pittsburgh, Pennsylvania; Chairman, Work Group on Managed Care, American Academy of Child and Adolescent Psychiatry.

InterCare, a multidisciplinary group practice with 15 psychiatrists (most of whom are child and adolescent psychiatrists) and an affiliated 50-bed child and adolescent psychiatric hospital, has been in the midst of this managed care transition. Having established itself as a community-oriented system providing comprehensive services, InterCare saw the changes being generated by the service shifts resulting from managed care as both opportunities and challenges. To our basic operations in fee-for-service and community mental health center work, we have added contracts with six or more utilization management companies and two major health maintenance organizations (HMOs). The latter makes us exclusively responsible for the children and adolescents of more than 290,000 HMO members. Because InterCare also provides adult services to part of this population, we can evaluate how managed care affects children and adolescents compared with adults. The following are areas I have found to be most significant.

There Is More at Risk

Managed care applies similar criteria to the management of adults and children. The appropriate diagnosis and effective treatment of psychiatric illnesses can have a profound effect on the child or adolescent making a transition into an adult, self-sustaining role, because young people are in the midst of dealing with so many developmental issues. The skillful treatment of an adjustment disorder or a single episode of depression not only relieves the suffering of the individual, but also often positively affects the way the family views and utilizes behavioral services and other costly medical resources. This positive effect is even more apparent with recurring and persistent problems (e.g., attention-deficit disorder, bipolar disorder, substance abuse). The suffering of the patients, their capacity to be cooperative partners in treatment, their utilization of resources, and their productivity will be affected for years to come.

The goal of treatment for children and adolescents is different than that for adults. Relief of symptoms and restoration of the previous level of functioning are insufficient. There must be a focus on restoration of developmental trajectory.

Children and Adolescents
Depend on a Support Network

The treatment of psychiatric illness and the restoration of a developmental trajectory can only be achieved when there is sufficient family, educational, and social support working in cooperation with medical treatment. The needs of children and adolescents and the limitations in their capacity to mobilize their own resources make them particularly vulnerable. Any rational system of behavioral health care must effectively evaluate and plan for the actual state of the support services. Many managed care criteria for inpatient treatment do not assign sufficient weight to these factors. The focus on reduction of the duration of inpatient treatment through telephone utilization management does not address the need for support and integration.

The Integrated Network of Self-Managing Teams

In contrast to utilization micromanagement, we need to develop innovative self-managing systems. Because of the importance of developmental and support network issues, child and adolescent behavioral services have always emphasized the team approach. This emphasis is most evident in high-intensity services (e.g., acute inpatient treatment or crisis intervention). In the new age of accountable health systems, the principles of effective teamwork must operate throughout the entire system and be particularly evident during the handoffs between different components of the system. These handoffs are best accomplished by clear definition of the mission, with anticipation of activities, services, and resource utilization. All components must be equally accountable and must welcome the feedback received from the different parts of the system (i.e., consumers, contractors, and colleagues). Quality management must focus on problem solving and continuous improvement in processes and systems. Team members must first be accountable to each other and then accountable to other system components. Staff members empowered to manage themselves through understanding the mission and goals of their component of the treatment can work as an effective team.

Some of the current external utilization management systems focus specifically on controlling the length of inpatient stay by withholding authorization for further treatment once the crisis stabilization goals have been achieved. A more effective behavioral health care system is responsive to the child's need to restore developmental trajectory. Such a system treats patients in a setting where resource utilization is efficiently managed but also where patients will receive treatment of sufficient duration and intensity to effectively modify psychopathology. That means, if possible, the avoidance of extended hospitalization and the encouragement of intensive outpatient and partial hospital treatment programs.

The Importance of Access

Dealing with multiple managed care companies can interfere with gaining access to competent assessment. When considering the needs of children and adolescents, there should be no limitation to the initial access to the system. Delaying treatment for a child increases the chance for developmental disruption and complicates the treatment process. Requiring that treatment be preauthorized by a primary care physician (particularly one with a financial incentive not to refer) adds an unnecessary step to the process of obtaining care. Inappropriately applied, such a requirement utilizes expensive health resources before analyzing the primary care physician's proper role in assessment. Parents, physicians, and school personnel need to be well informed regarding a simple process for obtaining access to the system. Research indicates that even when there are no financial barriers to seeking treatment, parents, pediatricians, and other primary care physicians fail to identify and refer children with significant psychiatric problems.

The efficacy and efficiency of a treatment system are enhanced not by keeping people out, but by understanding and shaping their expectations at the point of entry. By connecting them with the treatment resources best designed to respond to their needs and by helping them understand what they are expected to contribute to the treatment effort, the possibility of a positive outcome is greatly increased. Dissatisfaction frequently comes because of unmet expectations—not unmet needs. A cumbersome intake process designed from the viewpoint of the provider rather than the consumer increases frustration and dissipates motivation. Ineffective treatment often relates to a failure of commitment on the part of families and patients to an ongoing process of outpatient treatment and family systems change.

The Importance of Innovative Programs

23-Hour Observation

Some adolescents precipitate a destructive crisis as a way to avoid a sense of helplessness and to call attention to their need for help. If the crisis is handled through a routine inpatient psychiatric admission, the parents, the patient, the school, and the involved professionals all expect a hospital stay of 7–21 days. The family and school anticipate the relief of not having to worry about the problem for a period of time; the patient bonds with the inpatient staff and the peers in the milieu; the hospital chart and bill start to grow. Reversing this process is often very difficult and generally results in frustration. If, instead, when the patient presents for treatment, generally in crisis and late at night, the intervention is framed as an observation limited to less than 1 day, there is a marked change in perspective. During that day, the focus is on determining the appropriate setting for further diagnosis and treatment. This intervention has been successful in a highly integrated program in which the alternative programs (i.e., partial hospitalization, intensive outpatient therapy, in-home services) are immediately available and the handoff is smoothly executed. A key is that neither the patient nor the parents are allowed to settle into the hospital, and the hospital allocates no more resources or paperwork than is necessary to determine the appropriate treatment setting. Of course, if hospital treatment is appropriate, then the patient smoothly moves into the regular inpatient program.

Supplementary Intensive Programs

Although there has been a substantial decrease in the amount of inpatient psychiatric treatment for adolescents and children, this decrease is because managed care criteria establish that inpatient treatment is necessary only in situations of dangerousness, not because children and adolescents and their families are healthier and, therefore, need fewer services. Although an excessive amount of resources was allocated to inpatient treatment, many patients were helped through these intensive, focused services. The demands on the modern family make family members less able or willing to commit the resources of time, emotional energy, and modest financial payments. Therapists working in our full-risk HMO system are often in the position not of limiting services, but of encouraging families to take advantage of additional outpatient sessions. The demands of work and activity schedules, the $20 copayment, and the expectation for changes in the family system are powerful impediments to families availing themselves of the intensity of treatment needed to reestablish a child's healthy psychological development. For many patients, there can be significant benefit in therapy focused on short-term objectives, episodic family systems treatment, and appropriate use of medications. These are not sufficient, however, to deal with the serious problems encountered by the families of many children and adolescents. More appropriate treatment requires the development of innovative programs that are carefully evaluated in terms of efficacy and cost. The following are some possibilities.

Partial hospital programs.   When a child or adolescent communicates his or her distress through a crisis of dangerous behavior or cannot be maintained in the customary peer group settings at school, the patient and the family often need the intensity of daily, multimodal therapy past the time when the patient requires 24-hour supervision and nursing care. The crisis of a suicidal gesture of low lethality or a serious physical confrontation at home can be stabilized through a hospitalization for crisis intervention of several days. Moving all of these patients directly to outpatient treatment can safely manage the crisis and make the utilization statistics look good, but the substantial decrease in intensity of treatment, combined with the family's and the patient's patterns of minimization and denial, seals over the underlying conflict and perpetuates the psychopathology.

Partial hospital programs, particularly those integrated with an inpatient unit, can continue to utilize the tension mobilized by the crisis. A 6- to 8-hour intensive treatment program 5 days a week, with parents structuring the patient's evening and weekend time, keeps the focus on the therapeutic process and minimizes the distraction of other activities being used as a defense. These programs reduce the regression sometimes promoted by hospitalization and can be delivered with some reduction in cost. Keeping these programs closely associated with inpatient units is important so that there is not a break in the continuity of treatment between the crisis intervention phase and the ongoing therapeutic phase. A close association also permits brief rehospitalization if the patient did not have sufficient time to stabilize in the initial hospitalization or if uncovering of disturbing psychological material again precipitates a dangerous situation. There can also be a transition to the step-down intensive outpatient evening programs with group therapy, therapeutic activities, and individual and family therapy. This model of intensive partial hospital treatment may be a viable alternative for the patients who previously would have received and benefited from a 30- to 60-day inpatient stay.

Some issues create problems for this high-intensity, short-term partial hospital treatment model. If it is to be used for patients who would in the past have been hospitalized, the cost per day is still substantial because of the required investment of professional time. Evening programming and sleeping facilities do not account for half of the cost of a hospital day. The short length of stay creates a problem of turnover and variability of census that makes establishing a strong therapeutic milieu difficult. The actual demand for such services in a population group is low enough that a substantial population of perhaps more than a quarter-million people is required to maintain a viable program in a managed care environment. It is also hard to maintain the patients' and the families' investment. Problems of transportation and the requirement for family involvement sometimes lead to families' desiring discharge before this phase of therapy is actually completed.

Adjunctive programs.   Managed care, with its increased focus on therapeutic efficiency, challenges us to be innovative about how to generate greater therapeutic gain with fewer professional resources. Alcoholics Anonymous, the prototype mutual help group that is an essential rather than an adjunctive component of drug and alcohol treatment, has taught us the benefits of peer support, psychoeducational programs, and structured continuing-recovery plans. With adolescents, it is often the families who need to make significant changes. A mutual help group for parents of young people with alcohol and drug problems—Parents of Teens Addicted to Drugs and Alcohol (POTADA)—in the Pittsburgh area helps parents face their denial and enabling behavior. Families who are not ready to face the responsibilities of therapy can be referred to such groups. In that setting, they begin to understand the therapeutic process and prepare themselves for effective participation.

Children with Attention-Deficit Disorder (CH.A.D.D.), a national organization for families, is a vital part of treatment for families whose children have attention-deficit disorder. The support provided by CH.A.D.D. is especially important when there are limits on the number of outpatient sessions. These self-directed parent meetings and lectures go a long way toward helping parents understand the disorder, have appropriate expectations, and accept medication as a component of the treatment. They are invaluable in educating school personnel and in advocating for appropriate educational services and policies. Families participating in CH.A.D.D. require fewer outpatient sessions and can be better partners in treatment.

School-based services.   Schools are often children's most stable and responsive environment, and teachers and other school personnel are their most consistent and involved caregivers. In Pennsylvania, the statewide Student Assistance Program provides early and effective intervention for children at risk. Supplemented by school-based crisis intervention, referral, and therapeutic support programs, schools can be a location for early intervention and continuing therapeutic endeavor. InterCare provides school-based services through Education Prevention Intervention Consultants (EPIC), a program of school-based mental health personnel who are employed by our system and paid for by the schools.

The availability of such a program makes a crucial difference for an adolescent leaving a hospital after a 10-day stay for serious depression. The school counselor vividly remembers the student's suicidal statements. The teachers cannot imagine how someone so seriously ill as to require psychiatric hospitalization just a little over a week ago is now back in their classes. The student is frightened and uncertain about his or her own adjustment. An on-site mental health professional (located in the school district) who works with the hospital team is invaluable in helping the school to be a continuing therapeutic environment, in supporting the adolescent, and in ensuring that the transition to outpatient therapy works smoothly.

The EPIC professionals also work to prevent relapse by helping youngsters and families who are having difficulty accepting recommendations for psychiatric evaluation or who are becoming resistant to continuing in their outpatient treatment. They function as daily consultants to the school personnel who make up the student assistance team. Although there are many programmatic and administrative complexities in the establishment of such programs, school-based programs may be the most cost-effective intervention in the hectic lives of overstretched families. It is very hard to get children to come to an outpatient office or clinic, particularly during the day. Taking the therapy to them is a model that deserves evaluation.

Summary

Two decades ago, many children were denied necessary public education and treatment because they were "not appropriate" for selective educational and therapeutic settings. Federal and state right-to-education legislation and the growth of consumer-responsive psychiatric services broadened the accessibility of these settings. Now, managed care companies are saving money by changing "not appropriate" to "does not meet criteria." The provider community responds with appeals and protests. There must be broader access to care, but there will not be more money. The challenge is for creative providers to work in partnership with managed care companies to rethink our service delivery systems and to deliver effective, efficient treatment in innovative ways.

✣ 6 ✣

Drugs and Alcohol

The Managed Care View

CHIP SILVERMAN, PH.D., M.P.H.[*]

Credibility and legitimacy in the substance abuse treatment field were finally achieved in the 1970s, when insurance companies began reimbursing for such treatments. Unfortunately, the insurers were positively biased toward inpatient treatment, reimbursing at 80%–100%, and negatively biased against outpatient treatment, reimbursing at 50% or not at all. It was the insurance industry that also set the 28-day fixed length of stay that became the standard of alcohol and substance abuse treatment providers.

In 1981, 17 "cocaine hospitals" opened in Los Angeles within a 6-month period. These facilities charged anywhere from $5,000 to $30,000 per month and recommended an average of 8–9 weeks' stay. The insurance companies reimbursed handsomely.

By the middle to late 1980s, billions of dollars were spent nationally on inpatient chemical dependency treatment, despite a total lack of data that

---

[*]Director of Chemical Dependency, Government Relations and Public Affairs, Green Spring Health Services, Inc., Columbia, Maryland; former director of the Maryland Alcohol and Drug Abuse Administration.

showed any differences in clinical outcomes between inpatient and outpatient treatment. Thus, fixed lengths of stay were clinically indefensible, and insurers and businesses turned to managed care and utilization review to contain the high costs of inpatient chemical dependency treatment.

Today, most of the cocaine hospitals in Los Angeles have either closed or are offering alternative modalities of outpatient treatment and are treating larger numbers of those in need. Change comes slowly, however, and as recently as 1991, a majority of inpatient substance abuse facilities in Maryland were still living in the past, and outpatient treatment alternatives were difficult to find.

A study was conducted in Maryland to ascertain the extent to which substance abuse treatment providers recommended outpatient treatment, when appropriate, as an alternative to inpatient care. An unbiased third-party research project was conducted to document the admission practices of Maryland's chemical dependency patient care facilities. The design employed was an independent evaluation of a clinical scenario by six experts nationally recognized in the field of substance abuse and chemical dependency treatment. The experts were requested to evaluate the scenario and recommend the most clinically effective course of care without consideration for cost. The scenario follows:

> The patient is a 35-year-old white male who is single and employed as a sleep lab technician. He lives alone but has family (father, married brother, and married sister) living in town, not too far away. He has been a beer drinker for more than 20 years. He usually drinks only with friends, going out to a bar with the guys on his nights off. Lately, however, he has been buying a six-pack now and then on his way home from work and drinking it alone at home during the course of a few hours (he works the night shift and usually gets home around 8:00 or 8:30 A.M.). This solitary drinking has bothered him because it is something he really seems to enjoy, although he knows it's "wrong."
>
> Other substance use history includes having tried pot a few times and having tried cocaine only once (snorted with a friend at the ocean last summer). He admits to having last used pot around 2 to 3 months ago. He has never been to any kind of treatment before, although he has seen advertisements on TV in the mornings after getting home from work. He has given thought to seeking help, because he was drinking while seeing the ads on TV. He knows that this just "isn't normal."

One month ago, he was involved in an accident that was his fault (he hit two other cars that were pulling out of a parking lot while he was coming around the corner). He had been to a bar a few hours earlier with friends, and the police officer smelled alcohol on his breath. He was arrested for driving under the influence. He found a lawyer who recommended that he get into "some treatment program as fast as possible." He hasn't had anything to drink for a month since the accident.

Independent assessment of this scenario resulted in all six experts recommending outpatient care as clinically most advantageous to such a patient.

These findings were compared with those collected as a result of presenting the same clinical scenario to several Maryland chemical dependency rehabilitation facilities. Researchers contacted the providers and presented the clinical scenario as a potential candidate for treatment services. These findings were different from those of the independent panel: only 24% of the contacted treatment facilities recommended any form of outpatient treatment.

In addition, other variations of interest were noted during the study. These variations related to the personnel who accepted the researchers' calls and gathered the clinical information and to the type of service provided to the callers. The job descriptions of the facility personnel who accepted the calls ranged from nurses and treatment counselors to employees who were called "preadmission counselors." A significant number of calls were referred by the clinicians and counselors to employees whom they called "marketing staff." Many who took the calls seemed to be very busy with other duties and somewhat hasty to encourage utilization of their facilities.

Sometimes the research callers were put on hold during their conversations, and it appeared that the facility personnel were involved in other conversations while attempting to answer questions and give instructions to the research callers. Some facilities had personnel who were more interested in marketing and selling the facility and who tried to get insurance information: this attitude was in contrast to that of nurses and counselors, whom the researchers generally found helpful and sympathetic. Several facility personnel read from scripts or prepared statements encouraging a visit to tour and/or to be admitted to the facility.

A summary of recommendations from the facilities follows:

Facility 1 recommendation.   Inpatient detoxification and then a 21- to 28-day inpatient stay. This recommendation was given after extensive inquiry into insurance coverage.

Facility 2 recommendation.   On-site assessment was encouraged with the indication that it would lead to a recommendation to an inpatient stay. The inpatient stay was said to be a fixed program of 28 to 30 days.

Facility 3 recommendation.   On-site assessment was recommended before admission. The research caller was referred to marketing personnel, who offered to pick up the caller/patient and bring them to the facility.

Facility 4 recommendation.   Immediate inpatient treatment was recommended, with a 30-day fixed length of stay, after a preliminary inquiry about insurance coverage.

Facility 5 recommendation.   An on-site assessment and tour of the facility were recommended before a strongly implied admission.

Facility 6 recommendation.   Insurance information, name, and telephone number were relentlessly sought, with strong encouragement for inpatient treatment.

Facility 7 recommendation.   This facility indicated that it only provides, and recommends, inpatient care.

Facility 8 recommendation.   This facility recommended an assessment and a 4-week stay and offered to help with legal problems and to "prepare" the patient for court.

Facility 9 recommendation.   Inpatient detoxification followed by inpatient or outpatient treatment was recommended. Inpatient treatment was encouraged because "treatment would look good legally."

These facility recommendations are not uncommon from the perspective of a utilization management reviewer. In contrast, the physician reviewer evaluates each request for care individually, and the decision regarding the medical necessity of the requested level of care and treatment plan is based on the unique clinical information available. A careful examination of the clinical information, in the context of the publicly available, appropriate criteria for treatment, helps clarify the level of care that can be certified as medically necessary and appropriate for this patient.

Residential treatment was recommended by the nine facilities noted. Criteria for residential treatment of substance abuse include the severity-of-need and intensity-of-service components of medical necessity, which must be documented for certification of admission.

In the clinical scenario above, the patient reported a long history of social beer drinking several times a week. A recent increase in drinking frequency, possibly approaching a daily basis, also was reported. No occupational impact was noted as yet. An automobile accident about a month before seemed to precipitate his search for treatment. The accident also encouraged 1 month of sobriety, making a detoxification program unnecessary. Severity-of-need criteria for residential treatment require a continued inability to maintain abstinence despite recent professional outpatient intervention. Because the patient's living environment is not reported as dysfunctional, and because he is not a danger to himself or others, the information available would not allow certification of his admission because of severity of need. Further clarification of an appropriate level of care emerges when considering the intensity-of-service criteria for residential treatment. No significant impairment in the patient's social or occupational functioning that might require an inpatient rehabilitative setting has been reported; therefore, according to intensity-of-service and severity-of-need criteria, certification for residential treatment cannot be made.

Utilization management tries to encourage the use of the appropriate levels of treatment. Many utilization management companies propose alternatives: " . . . we never say 'no' without also saying 'yes.' " When physician reviewers cannot certify one level of care, they always try to encourage facilities or patients to consider alternate levels of care as possibly being more appropriate for certification. In the above scenario, the clinical data seem to encourage consideration of an outpatient treatment program. A structured daytime treatment program, in concert with an Alcoholics Anonymous sponsorship, seems a logical recommendation, given the patient's night work and lack of outpatient treatment experience. An employee assistance program and family involvement might also be worth considering.

Physician reviewers routinely talk with professionals from treatment programs when conducting certification reviews. But, with the appropriate authorization from the patient, some reviewers talk directly to patients and their families at the request of either the facility or the patient. In these cases, the reviewers try to educate the consumers of care about the reviewers' individual policies and about their certification functions. If asked, some physician reviewers will clarify why denial of care at one level was made, always following with a statement about the potential for approval of care at another, more appropriate, level.

Provider and patient expectations about the level of care desired are often different from the level of care that a physician reviewer can certify. Several utilization management companies have, from their inception, made their criteria for certification publicly available. Reviewers take the time to explain to facility staff, patients, and their families how the criteria relate to the presenting situation. Most utilization management companies provide, on request, a second opinion within 24 hours; when disagreement occurs, the providers are always encouraged to do what is clinically indicated from their perspective and to use an appeals process. The appeals process involves subsequent review of the written record of treatment provided by the facility or provider; documented medically necessary care can be certified on appeal.

Utilization management companies professionally consider each call and letter from providers and patients. An attempt is made to answer the questions raised with an explanation based on the specific clinical information available.

Over the last 4 years in Maryland, there has been an increase in non-inpatient treatment alternatives for patients with substance abuse problems. Utilization management companies believe in a spectrum of services along the outpatient-to-inpatient continuum. They have encouraged consideration of the appropriate level of care by individualizing each patient review. Providers have responded to the need for outpatient treatment with creative and diverse treatment modalities. Intensive day and evening programs are now available across Maryland, in both the private and public sectors, so that treatment can be tailored to the patients' work and home schedules. Utilization management firms continue to work with providers and patients in their intensive review processes to ensure an individualized review for each request for care.

Further research is necessary about specific treatment outcomes resulting from various treatment settings and modalities, especially those in the private sector. Only then will the most beneficial level of treatment become clear to providers, patients, and payers. Until such time that specific patterns of substance abuse have been shown to benefit from specific treatment protocols, substantial variation in treatment recommendations, such as that reported in the case presented above, will likely continue. In the interim, utilization management programs can help to ensure that each patient is certified for the most appropriate level of service that the available clinical information indicates.

The Clinician's View

SHELDON I. MILLER, M.D.[*]

In order to describe what is currently happening to the chemical dependency delivery system (or, for that matter, to consider its future), it is important to explore its history. The recent history of the system is brief. Many aspects of the system's development made it vulnerable—virtually from its inception—to the pressures of the present and to the changes likely to occur in both the immediate and the more distant future. Many of the factors critical to producing both past and future changes can be placed into two categories. The first category contains factors that could be described as either scientifically or economically valid, or both. The other category contains factors that must be described as unjustifiable—

---

[*]Director, Stone Institute of Psychiatry, Northwestern Memorial Hospital, Chicago, Illinois; Lizzie Gilman Professor and Chair, Department of Psychiatry and Behavioral Sciences, Northwestern University Medical School, Chicago, Illinois.

that is, they represent age-old prejudices and stigmas. Both the just and the unjust factors have been operative for years and are now magnified by the development of managed care.

For a moment, let's look at the history of treatment for chemical dependency and then, with the stage set, look at the legitimate and the problematic features of managed care regulation from this historical vantage point.

Modern abstinence-oriented treatment developed in the United States emphasized the problems of alcoholism and was only later adapted to treating other addictions. Although many schools of thought have contributed to our current understanding of addiction treatment, there are two that I believe have had a major influence on how things have developed. Both Alcoholics Anonymous (AA) and other more recently developed self-help groups, along with psychoanalytic theory and psychodynamic and psychoanalytic psychotherapy, have been influential in shaping the current treatment system.

One school of thought—the psychoanalytic—was important in a negative way. It defined addiction as a symptom and failed at first to recognize that a disease process was operative. The initial insights of the father of psychiatry, Benjamin Rush, were forgotten by the inheritors of his tradition. The 12-step groups (with AA being the most prominent) were led primarily by nonphysicians yet embraced the concept of addiction as a disease.

Because of the basic difference in the approach to the patient that resulted from the theoretical divergence, a wide gap developed between the advocates of the two positions, and treatment grew under the watchful eye not of psychiatrists but of non–medically trained individuals. The so-called Minnesota model of abstinence-oriented addiction treatment was nurtured by individuals who had little understanding of other psychiatric disorders and their relationship to addictive disorders. These individuals also began by building a program that was psychoeducationally based but was not developed within a scientific tradition of research and evaluation. Much of the content was determined by what had been helpful to others who had been successful in their own recovery and who sincerely believed that there was no better way to achieve sobriety. Physicians joined the effort, but many involved in the treatment community supported the approach without fostering scientific inquiry.

Some were interested in the outcome of treatment and began to ask questions. Ultimately, good research began, but throughout the inquiry the principal treatment was inpatient based, fixed in length, and non-psychiatrically directed or oriented.

The stigma surrounding these patients and those providing treatment helped influence the creation of a treatment system that existed primarily outside of the traditional medical system. For many years, the stigma played a large part in keeping the addicted person from being a benefactor of the expanding health insurance industry. Those who could pay out of pocket could sometimes find "quiet" (i.e., private and highly confidential) treatment, but for most people little such treatment existed. Not many years ago, this situation began to change. Through the efforts of devoted individuals, recovering and nonaddicted as well as lay and professional, insurance policies began to cover treatment for addiction and to provide expanded coverage for other psychiatric illnesses. Psychiatry and other branches of medicine began to understand that addiction was a disease. A high point was the American Medical Association's statement to that effect.

The availability of funding for care, coupled with the increasing demand for that care, led to an exponential development of new treatment facilities. There were two primary sources of the new treatment facilities. First, general hospitals were experiencing a decrease in demand for general medical and surgical beds. There was great resistance to closing licensed beds, and new sources of patients were sought. Addicted patients who had previously been stigmatized and unwelcome were now welcomed into hospitals.

The second and largest source of new beds was the building of free-standing hospitals dedicated to the treatment of addicted persons and, at times, psychiatric patients. Although some of these institutions were built by not-for-profit organizations, the greatest source was the growing for-profit chains, which often were a part of a larger, for-profit health care corporation. Although many of these companies were ethical and attempted to admit only patients who truly needed inpatient care, there was a large and significant group that seemed to be in the business to maximize profits regardless of the needs of the patients. Because physicians needed to be involved in each admission, questionable ethics governing some of the activities of these doctors contributed to the problem.

Unfortunately, the inpatient treatment approach was partially governed by a belief that a successful attack on the denial system of an addicted person required a treatment period of a fixed length. This belief resulted in little true individualization of treatment and, when coupled with the belief that most—if not all—of the symptoms seen could be explained by the addictive process, led to infrequent use of thorough psychiatric evaluation. This approach often produced outcomes that were both unfortunate for the patient and expensive. Patients failed to get well in the addiction setting because coexisting disorders went unrecognized. Longer stays resulted because the addiction failed to improve. Once the patients were discharged, relapse was more likely to occur in the face of an untreated psychiatric disorder. Finally, a psychiatric hospitalization might be required to treat what should have been attended to in the first place.

There was little motivation for anyone to question the almost exclusive use of inpatient treatment. At the time, persons who did try treatment in an outpatient setting were often not reimbursed by third-party carriers. Patients often had to pay themselves and had to do so in advance. Operators of hospitals did well financially. Because the treatment was primarily nonmedical, higher-paid medical professionals were not used. Medications for conditions other than detoxification were frowned upon. All of these factors reduced cost and maximized profits. Management of the system tended to be antipsychiatric; therefore, the idea of having a second psychiatric diagnosis that might interfere with treatment and outcome was not considered. Often the major provider of service was a nonmedical addictions counselor whose orientation and training simply did not incorporate an awareness of the prevalence of coexisting psychiatric disorders. The system generally was theoretically driven, not empirically governed. Admissions grew with strong marketing efforts stimulating demand.

New types of inpatient services proliferated. The "patient" in these services was not the addicted person, but rather someone associated with the addicted person. Inpatient beds became available for family members, who were told that the only way to recover was by spending time in an inpatient program. Obviously, inpatient treatment was not universally required of families, but it was frequently offered and encouraged.

Thus far, I have described the development of the most prevalent form of addiction treatment. That is the abstinence-oriented Minnesota model of addiction treatment first developed for alcoholism. Two other major types of treatment have also been developed; one is abstinence oriented and the other is not. The therapeutic-community movement had as its target population primarily narcotic-addicted people who wished to pursue an abstinence goal. The other approaches to this same population were the replacement therapies, exemplified by methadone maintenance.

Much could be said about these two important treatment approaches, but when considering the effect of managed care on the treatment system, these programs have been minor players. Many, and for a while nearly all, methadone maintenance programs were in the public sector and therefore subject to a different group of pressures. Many therapeutic communities also were in the public sector; and although many were not, they did not account for the dramatic expansion of services described above. I will not try to analyze the effect up to this time of managed care on these programs. I will say, however, that as time progresses, these programs, too, will clearly be of interest and will be looked at as candidates for managed care attention.

In concluding this discussion of the pre–managed care state of affairs, I think it would be helpful to give a brief account of what a typical patient entering a fixed-length program might experience.

Let us assume that our patient is a 35-year-old married father of two. He has been drinking since he was in college, but over the past 2 years his wife and, most recently, his employer have become increasingly concerned over his erratic and undependable behavior. He drinks daily, spending most evenings consuming alcohol and having little to do with either his wife or his children. Absences and decreased productivity are raising questions at work. He is depressed, irritable, and emotionally unpredictable with family and friends.

The patient's wife has seen advertisements for addiction treatment programs on television and has contacted one that encouraged her to bring her husband in to be evaluated. She is told to be prepared to admit him. She is successful in getting him to agree to an evaluation. When they arrive, they are interviewed by an addiction counselor and told that admission to the hospital program is the only thing that will help. The next day he is seen by a physician for a history and physical examination.

Detoxification is begun, and because the patient's mental status is relatively unaffected, he enters the ongoing group program. Although a treatment team (including nursing staff) and the admitting primary care physician meet, basically the outcome of the treatment team meeting is to direct the patient to the psychoeducational group program. His wife is enrolled in the ongoing family program. Individual counseling occurs twice a week with his primary counselor, and he briefly sees the doctor on daily rounds. Attendance at self-help programs is a necessary part of the program. The patient progresses through the program with periodic reevaluation of progress toward sobriety but no evaluation of his mental status. Discharge occurs about 1 month later, with aftercare consisting of a recommendation for daily self-help groups and biweekly attendance at aftercare groups. The wife is encouraged to attend her own self-help program.

This, then, is the stage onto which managed care came. It did not come alone, however. There was treatment outcome research literature culminating with The Institute of Medicine report. The report cast doubt on the primacy of the inpatient treatment setting as being most effective for delivering the type of care described above. In the report, the outpatient setting emerged as an equally viable and much less expensive setting in which to carry out treatment.

Much of the effect that managed care has had on chemical dependency treatment, therefore, is in areas where there were and are supporting scientific data. The previously mentioned Institute of Medicine report, as well as various research projects funded by the National Institute of Alcohol Abuse and Alcoholism and described in its reports to Congress, contains suggestions for changing the treatment setting from inpatient to outpatient.

Research on the treatment setting is not the only research that has supported the managed care approach to treatment. Two other lines continue to influence the process. There is increasing awareness, stimulated by the epidemiologic catchment area studies, that conservatively one-third (or less conservatively, more than one-half) of individuals with chemical dependency also have a second significant, non-drug-related psychiatric diagnosis. Obviously, this complicates the diagnosis and treatment. The fixed-length program with little psychiatric involvement, incomplete evaluation, virtual prohibition against any psychoactive medication, and little consideration for comprehensive aftercare planning could not continue unchanged in the face of hard scrutiny.

The other line of treatment research that has influenced the managed care field is the realization that addiction is a multifaceted diagnosis and that there are subsets of individuals who need to be described and differentiated in the treatment planning process. Although this research is far from definitive, differences among patients exist (even though they are yet to be fully clarified), and even now these differences must be evaluated and considered.

What has happened to the system, then, as a result of managed care? It is important to first define managed care, because there are two types that operate differently. First is the true health maintenance organization (HMO) approach with a closed, defined group of providers to whom the patient must go for all care. These programs have very often failed to provide acceptable care in any setting. The benefits tend to be poor and restrictive and at times ignore what is medically known in favor of simplistic and immediate savings. In many of these cases, there is not simply a reduction of the use of expensive care—there is next to no care. Patients are forced to seek help in the public sector—a system that is itself marginal and barely able to deal with those persons lacking sufficient resources. It seems as if some of these HMOs have taken advantage of the public's denial that addiction could happen to them and of the stigma that still is operative in our society. Money is saved while individuals go untreated. In addition, the stigma prevents an outcry that would be immediate if similar restrictions were put on patients with terminal, recurring cancer. Although this is a common situation, it is hardly universal; some HMOs are responsible and moral providers of care. These HMOs provide thorough evaluations using appropriate professionals and make available a spectrum of care.

The other type of managed care might better be called management of care. Here we are dealing not with controlled, direct provision by the company itself, but rather with management of the use of the benefits in a person's health care benefit package. There is some sorting out of who can provide care, as well as concurrent review of that care. The managed care companies that specialize in mental health and substance abuse generally are contractors with businesses or insurance companies that "carve out" these services from the rest of their health benefits. Again, as is true of HMOs, some of these companies are responsible and concerned, whereas others have no motivation or concern for anything but profit. The ethical companies attempt to ensure comprehensive evaluation of each patient and direct the care accordingly. Certainly, reduction of cost is important, but protocols exist that attempt to direct patients to effective treatment for their individual needs. Health care plan benefits are limiting factors for even the best management group and are, unfortunately, often limited not only by false economic assumptions, but also by stigma and lack of understanding.

The unethical managers restrict care even in the face of adequate benefits. The single driving force is maximizing profits. Decisions are not made with the patient in mind or on the basis of established protocols. They are arbitrary and pay little attention to the individual evaluation or to the available research.

The impact on the health care system of all of the above managed care activities has been dramatic. The effect on patients has varied, depending on the ethics of the managed care organization. The system has undergone a massive reduction of the number of inpatient beds for fixed-length programs. In a very few years, some large for-profit chains have reduced the number of chemical dependency beds by over half, and all providers who had such beds have had a similar and at times even more dramatic reduction. At the same time, there has been a significant increase in ambulatory programs and in partial hospitalization units. Whereas most detoxification was done previously in hospital beds, much is now done in outpatient settings, a procedure that is supported by recent research. Remaining inpatient services are now used only for the complicated patient, who is increasingly characterized as dually diagnosed (i.e., someone who requires both addiction services and treatment for other psychiatric disorders). Often these psychiatric disorders are the principal reason for admission, which is to an acute psychiatric unit with a staff trained in addictions as well as in general psychiatry.

Although some mourn the passing of the old treatment approaches, the changes described here are supported by available research. Companies characterized by fairly administered managed care, a willingness to settle for reasonable profits, an interest in delivering a quality product, and maintenance of an interest in the well-being of the patient are stimulating a welcome change in the delivery of addiction services to the uncomplicated addicted patient and to the dually diagnosed patient. Better and more comprehensive evaluations are being done, unnecessary hospitalizations are being avoided, treatment planning is comprehensive, and treatment for all of the problems needing attention—including psychiatric disorders requiring medication—is being given. The process has forced the field to develop a spectrum of services previously unavailable when there was no economic incentive to provide care in lower-cost settings. All these advantages and progress exist, however, only when dealing with ethical managed care organizations.

When care is unreasonably withheld, illness and suffering are fostered. In their pursuit of cost containment, the unscrupulous managed care organizations are aided by the stigma associated with addiction. The ethical managed care organizations attempt to find a reasonable balance of care, cost, and quantifiable outcome. Herein lies the challenge and the opportunity for ethical managed care organizations and professional providers. Continued outcome research using the tremendous data bases being developed should allow the scientists to answer questions about the efficacy of their differential treatment approaches. Some managed care people are gathering data that have enough detail to help answer the question of what is best for which addicted individual with what characteristics. This is a triple-win situation: for the company, for the scientist, and—most importantly—for the patient. If, however, the stigma associated with addiction is allowed to serve in the interest of cost containment with decreasing benefits in future health care plans, all will be losers.

Section III

Providers of
Clinical Services

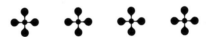

The Role of the Psychiatrist

The Managed Care View

ANTHONY F. PANZETTA, M.D.[*]

Managed care brings a new element into the mental health marketplace that will have a profound impact on the role of psychiatry. The element is competition. Psychiatry has not been required to operate in a true marketplace, where the forces of supply and demand shape the characteristics of the service offered and where competition sets the financial agenda. In a competitive marketplace, the psychiatrist's role in managed care will be largely "market driven." This is in sharp contrast to the traditional role of the physician, developed over many years of working in a relatively noncompetitive environment. The role of the psychiatrist in the "old" environment was set by personally chosen practice patterns, great autonomy, predictable financial security, and professional stan-

[*]President and Chief Executive Officer, TAO, Inc., Philadelphia, Pennsylvania; former Professor and Chairman of the Department of Psychiatry, Temple University Medical School, Philadelphia, Pennsylvania.

dards. Clearly, the managed care environment will be experienced as a "take away" in all but the professional-standards component.

A managed care company with which I am familiar had been developing standards for day-to-day operations as part of an extensive "quality management" initiative. Each department of the company was asked to establish at least five measurable objectives that would elevate the quality of activity in that department. The psychiatry department's response was to focus not on its own internal activities, but on the activities of other company clinical components. It was clear that the psychiatrists saw themselves as guardians of the quality of service provided by others but had difficulty focusing on their own internal practice characteristics. I present this anecdote as an example of a professional-entitlement world view that is largely shared by physicians in general. It is a perspective that has been honestly acquired through an educational process and subsequent work experience that emphasized the physician's role as "captain of the ship," or "ultimate authority."

The managed care environment has a different culture, and that culture will largely shape the role of psychiatry in managed care. It is the culture of business, where role function is determined on the basis of cost-benefit analysis rather than professional entitlement. The psychiatrist in managed care ultimately will perform those functions that only the psychiatrist can perform or those functions that the psychiatrist can perform cost-effectively compared with other persons performing the same function. It is a culture of competition and heightened cost consciousness.

For psychiatrists who are prepared to enter this new culture, there will continue to be gratifying work, professionally, ethically, and economically. But it will require a sea change in attitude and perspective. The essence of psychiatric practice (i.e., what goes on between a patient and a doctor) will continue to be shaped by the profession. Where practice is driven by scientifically supported evidence or supported by the consensus of the profession, there should be little change. That is what I referred to previously as "professional standards." It is the surrounding environment within which the psychiatrist works that will be different.

Clearly the trend will be toward group practice arrangements wherein a further differentiation of function occurs. Many managed care companies prefer to contract with group practices because they can thereby access multiple subspecialties in one setting and can also simplify the contracting and quality assurance system requirements (i.e., one contract and one system to cover the entire group). As a result, there will be a corresponding trend toward salaried positions rather than the current fee-for-service model. Provider groups will need to have predictable cost centers in order to bid successfully on contract opportunities. One way to accomplish this kind of stability and competitiveness is to move toward a salary-based budget.

Currently, psychiatrists develop their practices largely through their own individual efforts. They develop relationships with colleagues and with potential referral sources, and they count on a certain amount of word-of-mouth promotion. Their skills and their professional manner create what we can call their "professional image," and these elements determine the flow of patients into their practice. Competition between same-specialty physicians is played out in this professional-image marketplace. To some extent, the flow of patients to psychiatrists currently in group arrangements or in hospital-driven practices is not exclusively driven by professional image. These psychiatrists will not experience managed care as so great a dislocation.

The managed care environment is marked by much less opportunity for choice by patients. In all of the scenarios intended to bring cost containment to health care, the constraint on patients' choice stands out. The economics promised by managed care are to a large extent realized by control of the provider community—psychiatrists. In the managed care environment, psychiatrists become "manpower"—a component of a structured and managed delivery system. The more patient choice that is introduced into this environment, the less the system is under control.

Accordingly, patients will largely find their way into the practice of a psychiatrist because of assignment. Caseloads will more likely be standardized, and expectations for the outcome of care will be more explicitly defined. These efforts to bring standardization to psychiatric practice follow the usual tenets of business systematization. But psychiatric practice has been rarely systematized in this fashion, and so the changes will feel dramatic and intrusive.

As standardization takes hold, another shift will occur. In the mental health and substance abuse treatment arenas, therapy is delivered by at least three different professions: psychiatry, psychology, and social work. These three disciplines have drastically different historical legacies, professional identities, training, and expectations. In the current environment, these professions have competed for patients within the previously described professional-image marketplace and to some extent based on price. In the new environment of managed care, the flow of patients will be determined by the managers, and therefore the psychiatrist's market share will be determined by the laws of the market.

If three disciplines stake claim to a common therapeutic expertise (a prime example is psychotherapy), then the marketplace will use the discipline with the lowest cost, if one assumes equal efficacy as a result of care. When efficacy can be measured clearly, then these decisions are easier to make. But in the areas of mental health and substance abuse treatment, such certainty regarding efficacy is notoriously difficult to achieve. Consequently, there is a built-in tendency to assume equal efficacy and therefore go to the lowest-cost provider. Therefore, to compete adequately in the managed care marketplace, psychiatry must stake its claim to those components of the therapeutic process for which it is particularly efficacious and it must present compelling evidence of that efficacy.

Psychiatry has already experienced this shift in identity as a result of the community mental health movement. Given the cost constraints in the community mental health marketplace, the delivery systems that have developed no longer rest on a base of psychiatric manpower. Psychiatrists have been largely relegated to the role of prescribing drugs and managing pharmacotherapy. The exodus of psychiatrists from community mental health testifies to the power of a health delivery system driven by economic (business) principles. But the harbor to which many psychiatrists fled from community mental health, the private practice of psychiatry, is no longer a safe harbor. Managed care brings the same economic imperative to bear on this private harbor as was brought to the community mental health movement. It is now imperative to stay in the fray and to learn how to survive and perhaps even prosper.

I have used rather harsh strategic business terms deliberately because I believe that psychiatrists must come to grips with the fundamental shifts that are implicit in managed care. Glossing over these shifts will only compound the difficulties in adjusting to the new environment of managed care. Managed care is ultimately medical practice subjected to business strategy in the service of a competitive marketplace.

So we come to that place where the psychiatrist must step forward to say, "This is what I know, this is what I do, managed care cannot succeed without me, and this is why." I was asked to write this chapter because I am a psychiatrist and because I am the president and chief executive officer of a managed behavioral health care company. I believe that my being a psychiatrist has been very important in shaping the managed care "product" we attempt to deliver. The managed care that we deliver has been developed through the eyes of a psychiatrist.

I believe that psychiatrists bring the following extremely important strengths to the table:

1. A truly comprehensive health care perspective
2. Special expertise in the rapidly expanding area of biological psychiatry
3. Nearly exclusive competence in combined care using psychotherapy and pharmacotherapy (pharmacopsychotherapy)
4. A special and critical role in the treatment of seriously mentally ill persons

I believe that to succeed in managed care, psychiatrists must take the above strengths and join them with the following characteristics:

1. The willingness and ability to work in a true partnership with fellow professionals
2. The willingness to undertake a thorough reeducation about managed care and accept it with openness and an appreciation of its potential

Given the above strengths and characteristics, psychiatrists need not take a second position to anyone in the managed care clinical arena. The ultimate requirement in managed care is no different than it is in all of health care—treatment of individuals using the best knowledge, skills, and sensitivity. Managed care that fails to meet that requirement is not good managed care. This is an important point to understand. Many versions of managed care exist at this early juncture in its development. Some versions, particularly those that emphasize the denial of access to care, are destined to meet the ultimate reckoning at the hands of increasingly sophisticated quality oversight systems developed to monitor managed care activities. Rather than defaulting to others, psychiatrists need to enter the managed care environment and play a significant role in shaping that environment.

The Clinician's View

JOANNE H. RITVO, M.D.[*]

The facts are shocking: more than 30 million Americans are *without* health insurance, millions more are underinsured, and a third of our population has an identifiable but *untreated* mental illness (Santiago 1992). Our patients need our help. They need our support for a health care reform plan that includes universal access, high quality of the *appropriate* kind of care, and cost containment. Clinically, how can these features coexist in an era of managed care, and what special role do we psychiatrists play?

Psychiatrists are first and foremost physicians. Medically trained, and with special expertise in the diagnosis and treatment of all mental disorders, we alone among those in the mental health disciplines have expertise in both mind and body, in both the biological and psychosocial aspects of mental disorders. Medical school education and internship provide didactic as well as hands-on clinical experience shared only by other physicians. I believe that this experience of primary responsibility for the care of the bodies as well as the emotions of critically ill and dying individuals is so powerful that it is never forgotten; rather, it is integrated into our primary identity as physicians and as psychiatric physicians.

[*]Private practice in psychiatry, Denver, Colorado; Associate Clinical Professor of Psychiatry, University of Colorado Health Sciences Center, Denver, Colorado; Consultant, American Psychiatric Association Managed Care Committee; formerly Medical Director, Adult Unit, West Pines Psychiatric Hospital, Wheatridge, Colorado.

Residency training follows, producing psychiatrists who have more comprehensive supervised clinical training than persons in any other mental health discipline. They learn in outpatient clinics and locked psychiatric wards, in emergency rooms, and on medical and surgical units, where they provide psychiatric consultation and liaison for complex medical patients with emotional comorbidity or sequelae. During these formative years, they acquire the complicated armamentarium of skills for prescribing psychiatric medications—the treatments of choice for panic, obsessive-compulsive disorder, and other psychiatric disorders and clinically effective treatments for substance abuse and addictions. They learn the increasingly sophisticated psychopharmacology for schizophrenia, severe depressions, and bipolar conditions as well as treatment-resistant conditions. They learn to select one drug from many, to recognize and treat side effects, and to safely prescribe in the presence of concurrent medical illness and medications and for special populations, such as elderly persons.

As psychiatrists, we believed the specialty of psychopharmacology was ours alone. True, some nonpsychiatric physicians prescribe antidepressants or antianxiety medications and even lithium. But much more alarming to us is the recent lobbying effort by *nonphysicians* providing mental health care who want the legal authority to prescribe drugs. We do not see this as a turf battle but rather as an issue of the quality of patient care—of the patients' best interest. I cannot express it better than the American Psychiatric Association's English et al. (1992):

> We would not propose that legislative fiat, rather than years of additional supervised residency training, should entitle psychiatrists to perform coronary artery bypass surgery. Even though they are trained physicians, that is not where psychiatrists' expertise lies, and the patient would be at risk. (p. 1147)

English et al. questioned the disturbing assumption that, somehow, being granted "provider payment status by Medicare or other health insurers automatically confers parity of education, training, expertise, clinical experience, and, indeed, the authority to provide medical services" (p. 1147).

Psychiatrists remain the only physicians and the only mental health providers with both this expertise and the expertise to administer the cost-effective combination of psychopharmacology and psychotherapy. Even now, when advances in biological psychiatry unthinkable 20 years ago occur seemingly on a daily basis, psychiatrists teach and learn psychotherapy: cognitive-behavior, interpersonal, and group psychotherapy. It is deplorable that the expertise of psychiatrists as psychotherapists is so ignored and downplayed, although it has been demonstrated to be cost-effective and efficient.

A discussion of the special role played by psychiatrists in today's era of managed care and health care reform would be incomplete without noting their indispensable role as team leaders, triage physicians, and "traffic cops" in all settings of mental health care. They alone are appropriate to *direct* patient care, to recognize comorbid medical problems and ensure that they are not ignored during dangerously short hospital stays, and to oversee the somatic interventions of psychopharmacology or electroconvulsive therapy and their coordination with the psychosocial therapy.

Finally, the special role of psychiatrists in managed mental health care has evolved increasingly to include a specific, challenging, and at times frightening *responsibility* and *liability*: care for the very sickest and most dangerous psychiatric patients. This care occurs increasingly in less restrictive environments, in ever decreasing time frames, and with diminishing resources. We are told we must "manage" (sometimes barely) these sicker patients outside of a hospital setting. Yes, a continuum of partial hospitalization, residential treatment options, and outpatient follow-up for these patients should be in place, but frequently it is lacking.

It is my opinion (as a former medical director of an acute adult psychiatric unit) that the stress of caring for such patients under these circumstances is greatly underappreciated. Many psychiatrists with considerable talent for inpatient psychiatry have burned out and no longer accept acutely ill patients. They find that caring for these patients is too emotionally draining and time consuming for the reimbursement received. Psychiatrists must rapidly assess these patients' problems and delineate a treatment plan that must be implemented immediately. Additionally, the psychiatrist in charge must attempt to gain an alliance with a severely disturbed and disorganized patient who may be only marginally reconstituted when discharged to an alternative treatment site some few days later. As a result, the likelihood that the patient will pay his or her portion of the psychiatrist's fee decreases, while the chances for litigation increase. Yet the competitive down-pricing of psychiatric services continues, threatening our very livelihoods and incentive to care for these patients.

Under managed care, I fear that the stigma that has plagued psychiatrists and our patients for years may be increasing. Other mental health disciplines may gain some distance from this problem by referring to persons whom they see as "clients." But we, as physicians, call those we see "patients." In the current era, this practice may be backfiring; as managed care develops a "tier" system, it appears that only the most severely ill patients are referred to psychiatrists or allowed to continue in treatment with them (even though more experienced care providers frequently treat patients for shorter lengths of time). Unfortunately, both medical managed care gatekeepers and nonphysician mental health providers contribute subtly to this stigmatization ("You're not sick enough to see a psychiatrist"; "You don't have that big a problem or need medication"; "I'll refer you to a 'counselor' ").

Faced with this trend, psychiatrists suffer, but unfortunately, patients may suffer more, experiencing greater morbidity as more subtle conditions such as chronic hypomania or panic disorder go unrecognized and inadequately treated. Psychiatrists experienced in pharmacotherapy are more likely to appreciate the wider indications for the use of medication in a clinical situation. When nonpsychiatric physicians or clinicians fail to recognize such clinical signs or believe a nonmedical therapist can treat the patient "just as well," patients may be deprived of the most clinically effective and cost-effective treatment. Then, conditions that would otherwise respond to an appropriate combination of medication and psychotherapy continue, requiring longer, more costly treatment and resulting in increasing morbidity. The case of Mr. C. illustrates this problem:

> Mr. C. is a 40-year-old executive who is in the eighth month of his second course of weekly psychotherapy with a very experienced doctoral-level therapist. He has a lifelong pattern of inappropriate explosive reactions; chronic irritability; and rejection sensitivity; and, sometimes, acknowl-

edged depression. Although no significant legal difficulties have resulted, there have been many close calls with authority. No history of frank mania in the patient or his relatives was obtained, but he reports his mother as equally volatile and his brother as a polysubstance abuser.

Mr. C. was referred for psychiatric consultation after he overreacted to a perceived rejection by his girlfriend, and he became physical with her. Based on his irritability and volatility, as well as distractibility and psychomotor agitation, Mr. C. appeared at first visit to be suffering from an agitated depression or possible hypomanic state. He was begun on a trial of sertraline 50 mg/day. Within days, he appeared visibly calmer and reported significant improvement in mood and frustration tolerance; indeed, he said he felt better than he had in years. His girlfriend validated his improvement. He will be monitored for evidence of mania precipitated by the antidepressant. Had Mr. C. received an evaluation by a psychiatrist when he presented 3 years earlier, he could have been saved considerable pain and undue expense.

Other concerns for the psychiatrists (and yes, I certainly am not the first to state these concerns) center around the ever-increasing amount of time spent satisfying the demands of managed care for information: filing insurance forms, detailed treatment plans, and follow-up reports and spending time on the phone with reviewers justifying "medical necessity" for treatment. When the reviewer is not a psychiatrist, we receive the clear message that our time is less valuable than that of the psychiatrists employed by the managed care company. To date, this time has not been billable to insurance. Indeed, I literally have spent time spelling "hypokalemia" and explaining the life-threatening effects of low potassium while a reviewer slowly entered the data into her computer. Another psychiatrist would appreciate these medical complexities. Although this chapter is not devoted to fiscal issues per se, it must be noted that eventually our administrative costs will be passed on to patients.

Practitioners report that such experiences contribute to increasing feelings of impotence, disenchantment with our profession, and ultimately to burnout. Additionally, I believe this trend contributes significantly to the decline in the number of medical students choosing psychiatry as a specialty! The low morale and job dissatisfaction of their teachers impress them.

Additionally, patients frequently get caught in an enigmatic maze of managed care decisions. This so-called "Catch-22 effect" makes no clinical sense: if patients begin to reconstitute, they are discharged because the treatment is no longer "medically necessary"; if they do not reconstitute quickly, pressure is exerted for discharge because they are deemed "unresponsive to treatment" (Lewin and Sharfstein 1990). Practitioners observe that inadequate nonpsychiatric case management of patients can lead to early discharge, high readmission rates, and even suicide. Mismanaged managed care can be dangerous, but more frequently, it is disruptive to care and caregivers, as it was in Ms. D.'s care:

> Ms. D., 32 years old, is a brittle diabetic, previously diagnosed with chronic recurrent major depression and borderline personality disorder with frequent dissociative episodes. A childhood victim of incest by her father, Ms. D. was a true survivor of unimaginable horrors. She was not manipulative or gamey; when she took her insulin and did not eat, she wanted to die to escape the pain.
>
> After several brief hospitalizations within 18 months, Ms. D. made a near-lethal suicide attempt with her insulin and was found comatose. After stabilization, Ms. D. actually agreed to stay in the hospital to work on the terrifying memories that plagued her. She could not do this work as an outpatient. Her trust was insufficient and her fear too great.
>
> However, after 7 days, the managed care reviewer began to call me as well as this very suicidal patient every other day. She questioned the patient's daily progress, suicidality, and need for continued hospitalization although the patient was in a trancelike dissociative state. Her tenuous hold on reality and sense of safety were severely threatened. In short, she was being retraumatized by total strangers, a horrible reexperiencing of the intrusion of the worst kind by her father.

Psychiatrists with both inpatient and outpatient practices deal constantly with these stresses. There is a constant need to protect one's patients from such intrusions. In Ms. D.'s case, I believe the ultimate 30-day stay would have been significantly shortened without these violations. Such a situation should *not* happen! The *American Psychiatric Association Manual of Quality Assurance* has an entire chapter on protecting confidentiality of patient records (e.g., during phone reviews)—yet reviewers feel entitled to come into the hospital, phone the patient, and interject themselves into the treatment.

Protecting patient confidentiality appears to be a virtually impossible task with managed competition. A trend that particularly alarms me is the growing tendency of companies to request the "entire record"—including treatment "notes" and so forth—not just a treatment summary and medication record. I am told that this request is not legal in many states, but if the provider refuses to send the entire record (citing concerns about patient confidentiality), the insurance company may withhold payment, noting that the patient "signed a release."

Finally, the trend of utilizing provider networks poses problems for many psychiatric patients because these networks so disrupt continuity of care. In psychiatry, perhaps more than in any other medical specialty, our patients require continuity in order to make and sustain progress. Increasingly, we recognize the significant traumas—abuse, abandonment, neglect—sustained by our patient population. They lack trust. To require them to change caregivers each time an employer changes insurance companies is unconscionable and just bad medicine. That happened to Ms. E., a divorced teacher with severe unipolar depression, narcolepsy, and a chronic pain disorder. With a history of severe emotional and sexual abuse, she had such severe trust issues that she did not date for 5 years, fearing she would be retraumatized. Although she was able to work, her functioning was often marginal. She required multiple medications, a 1-week hospitalization when most suicidal, and twice-weekly psychotherapy for 2 years before she was stabilized. She now is seen every other week but requires two to three phone calls per week as she struggles to maintain connection, reality testing, and continuity. Recently, she and I were told that although she had made significant gains with me, she would need to select a new psychiatrist as I was soon to be an "out of network" provider. Without question, a forced change of therapist is detrimental to such patients, precipitating regressions and costly hospitalizations.

How has psychiatry coped with the problems and expectations raised by managed care? I believe an honest answer is, "We are trying to adapt." We are learning to document, objectify, and quantify. Psychiatrists are forming more group practices, although many resist the idea that solo practice may become outdated. Psychiatrists protest that our practices are already "lean and mean" and our overhead is as low as possible. However, our administrative costs are rising, along with the cost of malpractice insurance. Many practitioners I know are hiring office managers for the first time, a disturbing trend that reduces net incomes while ultimately increasing health care costs.

Additionally, increasing numbers of psychiatrists have joined with other mental health providers in order to market themselves to employers. Although many regret the diminished emphasis on psychotherapy in their practices, they reluctantly team up with nondoctoral-level therapists to comply with managed competition trends. Many of us believe this trend, if carried to an extreme, could destroy psychiatry as a medical specialty.

On a national level, the American Psychiatric Association has tried to be proactive. An "800" number was instituted to enable members to report managed care problems. Delegates from the managed care committee engage in dialogue with representatives of managed care, hoping to promote future cooperation and diminish adversity.

As we enter a new era of managed competition and health care reform, psychiatrists hope to retain our differential advantage. Although the shape of psychiatric practice is changing, I can only hope our core and complexity will be retained. I believe that if psychiatrists are reduced to biological diagnosticians and team leaders only, we will sacrifice the psychosocial aspect of the biopsychosocial model that drew most of us into psychiatry and eliminate the invaluable integration we alone offer patients.

I hope that universal health care will ensure mental health coverage for all, while focusing on our patients' needs for confidentiality, continuity of care, and some choice of providers. Patients with severe mental illness as well as character disorders must have an identified caregiver. As psychiatrists, we can urge that managed competition not "throw the baby out with the bathwater" by eliminating access to private practitioners altogether. There should also be a way for those who want more labor-intensive treatment to pay for and receive it. The rationale that psychiatrists will see the same patient at many strategic points in his or her life rather than for a sustained period of time is acceptable for many patients. However, this "pit-stop therapy" may be inadequate for some patients; their lives may require more of an engine overhaul. For our patients' mental health as well as our own, we must support reform that respects care constancy, adequacy, and reimbursement.

References

English J, Cutter J, Meyers N: Letters in the patients' best interests. Hosp Community Psychiatry 43:1147–1148, 1992

Lewin R, Sharfstein S: Managed care and the discharge dilemma. Psychiatry 53:116–121, 1990

Santiago J: The fate of mental health services in health care reform, I: a system in crisis. Hosp Community Psychiatry 43:1091–1099, 1992

The Role of the Psychologist

The Managed Care View

NICHOLAS A. CUMMINGS, PH.D., LITT.D.[*]

As the era of cost containment in mental health care continues to promote managed care, it is important to look briefly at the historical back-
drop against which the delivery system is evolving. Professional
psychology as a dispenser of clinical services was born in World War II
when General William Menninger made the decision to place personnel
trained in psychotherapy at battalion aid stations on the battlefield. Faced
with a shortage of draft-eligible young psychiatrists, he resorted to send-
ing clinically untrained psychologists to the School of Military Neuro-
psychiatry at Mason General Hospital and to giving them 60- to 90-day
training along with physicians who had just graduated from medical
school. Before World War II, there were two small groups of practicing

[*]President, Foundation for Behavioral Health, San Francisco, California; founding
Chairman and Chief Executive Officer, American Biodyne (retired), San Francisco,
California; President, National Academies of Practice; former President, American
Psychological Association.

psychologists. Members of the first group, though sometimes prominent (e.g., Theodore Reik, Sigfried Bernfeld), were more identified as lay analysts than as psychologists. The second group consisted of a handful of psychologists, mostly women, who worked with children (e.g., Nancy Bayley, Florence Mateer), often in very unlikely places (e.g., Columbus, Ohio; Carbondale, Illinois) in the nation.

After World War II, these psychologist pioneers were replaced by first a trickle, and then a steady stream, of veterans who sought doctoral training as clinical psychologists. Finding the early postwar training programs woefully inadequate, they obtained their significant clinical training off campus from congenial psychiatrists who also referred their overflow patients to these psychologists and then supervised them in their fledgling practices. These early psychologists eagerly emulated their mentors, an attitude that changed to confrontation and challenge years later when clinical psychology reached its adolescence. During the next several decades, psychology established itself as an autonomous profession, and it is now regarded as the penultimate mental health profession even though there are more psychologists than psychiatrists in independent practice.

Also during this time, the psychopharmacological revolution took place. As psychiatrists understandably gravitated to the biological therapies, psychology became identified as the premier psychotherapy profession. It was during this time that psychology made great strides in discovering more effective and efficient psychotherapies. The marketplace tacitly and comfortably accepted both biological and psychological therapies, and the war between psychiatry and psychology would probably have faded away were it not for psychology's decision to expand its frontiers to include hospitalization and medication privileges. Further, with the advent of managed mental health care, respective responsibilities and functions of the two professions became blurred, making managed care erroneously appear to be a psychiatry-psychology conflict. Actually, the conflict arises from the industrialization of health care. As is true in all industrialization, those who make and deliver the product (in our case, the practitioners, whether they are psychiatrists or psychologists) lose control over the product. As of this writing, organized psychiatry has ameliorated its original stance to managed care and is actively engaged in meaningful dialogue with it, while organized psychology continues its strident opposition. Predictably, psychiatry will have the greater influence on the future development of managed care. What, then, is the psychologist's role in the delivery of services in a managed care environment?

The brief initial period when roles were blurred has given way to the reestablishing of the psychiatrist's authority as medical director, while the preponderance of psychotherapeutic services are rendered by psychologists. The psychiatrist is firmly in charge of hospitalization on a team model, but hospitalization under managed mental health care is significantly reduced in favor of outpatient services. For every $4 million in reduction of inpatient costs, approximately $1 million is redirected into additional ambulatory care in which the psychologist is a significant participant. But managed care is more than the dispensing of mental health services: it is an integrated delivery system that has the potential to change markedly the manner and kinds of services rendered. An analysis of where managed care is heading reveals that psychotherapy will be delivered in a manner that restores some of the autonomy and control that are important to psychologists.

The first generation of managed care, of which almost every reader is now aware, involves telephone utilization review and limited benefits. The second generation of managed care, which is not as frequent but is growing rapidly, continues telephone utilization review and limited benefits but adds an unmanaged provider network administered through a negotiated, discounted fee for service. The third generation of managed care, which is just now beginning, is characterized by expansion of benefits. This expansion is made possible by networks of providers trained in managed care and time-shortened therapy techniques, with clinical case management of outpatient services as well as on-site hospital review, a defined continuum of care, and the inclusion of life-style management programs. Within this third generation everyone has heard of networks of "preferred providers." A new concept is emerging that goes beyond preferred provider to "prime provider," called "retained provider" in one progressive managed care company. Here is where the opportunity lies.

Retained providers are a group of practitioners who not only are able to deliver the wide range of services required, but also have demonstrated quality, efficiency, and effectiveness. These groups of retained providers will contract with the managed care firm to be responsible for all the care for a specified enrolled population—for a prospective reimbursement. Because the group has proven its quality, effectiveness, and efficiency, the managed care company no longer case-manages the group and only does "arm's-length" monitoring to ensure that services provided meet the contractual standards. Thus, the managed care company profits by saving the expense of case management, and the practitioners benefit by having their autonomy restored.

The group practices that achieve the status of retained providers will prosper in a climate of relative austerity. These groups will be multifaceted, able to perform the entire range of psychotherapy and life-style management services. They will be skilled in focused, targeted interventions and will know how to practice brief, intermittent psychotherapy throughout the life cycle. The group practice model called "the general practice of psychology," as first proposed 15 years ago by N. A. Cummings and G. R. VandenBos, is still relevant in this new arena, and farsighted psychologists are beginning to move rapidly in that direction on their own initiative. These are the psychologists who will not only survive but prosper as they meet the needs of society during an industrial health care revolution.

An organizational setting such as that provided by managed care makes possible extensive outcome research. Insurers have long been mystified by what we do as psychotherapists. They had no basis on which to question treatment decisions as to duration, intensity, or outcome. This situation is about to change.

For decades, psychologists conducting outcome research have pointed to the growing irrelevance of schools of psychotherapy; their research indicates that all schools embody some truth, but no one school embodies all the truth. They called for specific treatments designed to ameliorate specific psychological conditions. In my own writings, I have been particularly scathing, pointing out that psychotherapy is the only field of health where the patient receives the treatment the therapist was trained to provide, rather than the treatment that the patient's condition requires. In other words, whether one has a marital problem, a phobia, or a job problem, the patient receives the couch, the painting of pictures, or desensitization, purely on the basis of whether the therapist is a Freudian, a Jungian, or a behaviorist. This criticism is admittedly overdrawn, but the point still remains that too often all patients, regardless of presenting complaints, receive essentially the same treatment approach.

Working independently and on opposite coasts, S. H. Budman and N. A. Cummings reported research demonstrating that some conditions best respond to dynamic approaches, whereas others respond well to behavioral or systems approaches. However, most conditions respond best to specific, empirically derived amalgams of all schools of psychotherapy. The admixture varies with the psychological condition. Budman predicted an eventual "blurring" of the boundaries dividing the various approaches, whereas Cummings foresaw the "melding" of all the schools of psychotherapy into admixtures. Cummings also predicted that instead of keeping a patient in therapy for protracted periods until all problems and potential problems were resolved, the psychotherapist of the future would practice "brief, intermittent psychotherapy throughout the life cycle," not unlike the practice of all the health fields, which treat specific problems as they arise, with continuity for chronic conditions.

Now, in psychology's centennial year, many of the leaders in psychotherapy—after showing signs for several years of moving in that direction—are flat-out predicting psychotherapy "integration." Diverse clinicians representing a wide range of approaches are predicting not only integration, but also empirically derived, focused, targeted treatment of specific conditions, emphasis on brief and time-limited interventions, and accountability; some are even predicting treatment manuals. Managed care, through its ability to conduct outcome research on a large scale, will hasten psychotherapy integration, for standardization of the product is the propensity of all industrialization.

An effective, clinically driven managed care system concentrates not on saving money, but on clinical effectiveness, which ultimately achieves both efficiency and cost savings. This clinical effectiveness not only requires therapeutic skills that not all therapists possess, but also requires a shift in attitude on the part of the therapist.

Forms of brief therapy immediately come to mind. Effective, efficient psychotherapy is not necessarily brief therapy, although effective psychotherapy may be less time intensive than ineffective psychotherapy. Appropriate therapy is the least intrusive intervention necessary to do the job. For some patients, this may mean long-term therapy, but it is long term based on the patient's need, not the psychotherapist's ineffectiveness. In our own work in deriving specific, empirically tested therapies (see Cummings 1992), we regard the following statement as the Patients' Bill of Rights:

> The patient is entitled to relief from pain, anxiety, and depression in the shortest time possible and with the least intrusive intervention.

This Patients' Bill of Rights presupposes that the therapist will hone his or her skills to be able to fulfill these rights. It follows that the therapy of the future will be pragmatic, eclectic psychotherapy. Efficiency is clinically driven rather than driven by cost containment. It allows for intermittent therapy throughout the life cycle of the patient rather than one protracted episode intended to solve all problems for all time.

Less than one-third of psychotherapy in the future will be done on a one-on-one basis. This idea, which will be startling to most clinicians, will undoubtedly be the most controversial of our predictions. Individual psychotherapy, even when it is effective and efficient, is still labor intensive. It drastically limits the number of patients a therapist can see in a given day. This limitation would be acceptable if individual therapy were the best way to treat all patients. Recent outcome research, still in the preliminary stages, strongly suggests that what has been known for some time about alcoholic patients may be true for many other (if not most other) patients: a group program yields better therapeutic outcomes.

Patients with personality disorders, especially Axis II patients, do not generally respond therapeutically to the therapist (parental) transference. They defy authority, frustrate treatment by acting out between sessions, and are regarded as needing long-term treatment of as much as a decade or more. Inasmuch they defy parental (therapist) authority, those persons stuck in a perpetual mode of adolescent rage respond quite readily to the peer (group) transference. The peer pressure of the group can confront and control acting out in a manner that would not be accepted from the therapist. Because the number of persons presenting for treatment with these personality disorders is increasing, we predict that in the not-too-distant future, in effective delivery systems only 30% of psychotherapy will be one-on-one, whereas 70% will be focused group therapy and targeted psychoeducational programs.

Summary and Conclusions

Although the wide-open window of opportunity accorded psychologists a few years ago when managed care was just beginning is gone, there are still opportunities for practitioners not only to survive but also to thrive in the new environment. Psychologists who can prepare for this rapidly growing delivery system will find that managed care will actually increase the amount of monies allocated to outpatient care compared with inpatient care. Managed care will gravitate from preferred providers to prime (retained) providers, and those practitioners who can hone their skills and competencies will prosper.

A number of propositions designed to enable the psychologist to become a retained provider (thus restoring the professional autonomy lost to the preferred provider) have been presented. Psychologists need to prepare for the fact that managed care in some form will be the modal delivery system for universal health care, which is likely to be adopted this decade. Therapy will be pragmatic and eclectic, will favor the least intrusive and most appropriate level of care (such as outpatient psychotherapy versus unnecessary hospitalization), and will be focused and targeted throughout the life cycle. Psychologists will not only have to hone their skills, but also reexamine their attitudes.

Recommended Reading

Austad CS, Berman WH (eds): Psychotherapy in Managed Care: The Optimal Use of Time and Resources. Washington, DC, American Psychological Association, 1992

Bloom BS: Planned, Short-Term Psychotherapy: A Clinical Handbook. Needham Heights, MA, Allyn & Bacon, 1991

Budman SH, Gurman AS: Theory and Practice of Brief Therapy. New York, Guilford, 1983

Cummings NA: The emergence of the mental health complex: adaptive and maladaptive responses. Professional Psychology: Research and Practice 19:308–315, 1988

Cummings NA: Brief, intermittent psychotherapy throughout the life cycle, in Brief Therapy: Myths, Methods and Metaphors. Edited by Zeig JK, Gilligan SG. New York, Brunner/Mazel, 1990, pp 169–184

Cummings NA: The future of psychotherapy. Independent Practitioner 12:126–130, 1992

Friedman S, Fanger MJ: Expanding Therapeutic Possibilities: Getting Results in Brief Therapy. Lexington, MA, Putnam, 1991

Goldfried MR, Castonquay LG: The future of psychotherapy integration. Psychotherapy 29:4–10, 1992

VandenBos GR, Cummings NA, DeLeon PH: Economic and environmental influences in the history of psychotherapy, in The History of Psychotherapy. Edited by Freedheim DK. Washington, DC, American Psychological Association, 1992, pp 11–31

The Clinician's View

DANIEL J. ABRAHAMSON, PH.D.*
ALFRED A. LUCCO, PH.D.**

Managed mental health care crept into the practice of psychology over an extended period of time as a result of concern for the continuously rising cost of mental health services. Unfortunately, this concern came to be expressed as an accusation that clinicians would not monitor themselves and, hence, would keep patients in treatment unnecessarily. The history of psychology's response to this concern includes efforts at "self-control" through the development and popularization of short-term treatment methods and peer monitoring systems such as the National Register

* Administrative Director, The Traumatic Stress Institute, South Windsor, Connecticut; State and Federal Advocacy Coordinator, Connecticut Psychological Association; Consultant, American Psychological Association—Practice Directorate.
** Cofounder, The Center for Development (a multispecialty mental health group), Baltimore, Maryland; Associate Professor, School of Social Work, University of Maryland at Baltimore.

of Health Care Providers in Psychology and the peer review committees of local and state psychological associations.

One of the early and less direct attempts to control the rising cost of mental health services through legislation was the inclusion of more and more mental health professions in the aggregate of practitioners eligible for third-party reimbursement. This market device—inflation of supply rather than decrease of costs—resulted in increased costs due largely to the vast unmet demand for mental health services. This attempt at cost cutting was followed by limitation of benefits through precertification, utilization review, treatment plans, and aggressive inpatient monitoring (the major source of early cost-cutting success).

Currently, the management of mental health services has gone from utilization review to the establishment of networks of providers who work for lower fees and are willing to identify themselves with a short-term treatment philosophy and/or "in-house" service provision units operated by managed care companies. High-tech information processing systems are used to profile network providers and identify those whose pattern of service delivery is most in keeping with the treatment philosophy of the managed care company. These latest changes are affecting the social context within which psychologists practice through major shifts in the consumer experience.

It is the consumer's reality that defines the working context for the psychologist-patient relationship and the mutual role expectations. The structure emerging now—large managed care organizations controlling mental health services to very big populations across the country—involves a mode of control and referral quite different from the former process of reliance on gatekeepers, good friends, and professional advisers. Attempting to access mental health services today, many consumers face a myriad of obstacles. These restrictions range from denial of access to treatment to the requirement for frequent intrusive reviews of the ongoing treatment process. The result has been a deterioration of consumers' freedom of choice and psychologists' professional autonomy.

Psychologists participate in managed care in one of two ways: as solo or group practitioners with some managed care contracts or as the employees of an in-house treatment facility for a managed care company. Although similar elements affect both arenas, the impact on practitioners varies somewhat depending on how they participate in managed care.

This impact will be noted as we consider both the structure and the functions of managed care psychological practice.

Structure

The most rapidly changing element of structure is the relationship between the individuals involved in the health care transaction. The role expectations for both the psychologist and the client have changed, and a third role—management—has been added. Before this shift, the structure was one in which an expert (psychologist) was hired by a person in need (client) to achieve a resolution of a particular set of problems. Two elements of role expectation are noteworthy in this arrangement: 1) the psychologist works for the client, and 2) the psychologist by virtue of expertise and professional reputation is permitted to be an authority in determining the conduct of the helping transaction. Under managed care, there is a lack of clarity with regard to either element. For the private practitioner, there is a split between power and responsibility wherein the managed care company works to maintain decision-making power and to give the psychologist practitioner the ultimate responsibility for client well-being. When the psychologist is an employee, the structure looks more like an organizational chart, with the managed care company at the top (represented by a set of rules and guidelines for practice); the psychologist in the middle, representing the company's position in the best possible manner and making decisions according to policy; and the client at the bottom, with little or no freedom of choice or decision-making power.

A major consequence of this shift in structure has been the erosion of professional autonomy. Such an erosion is, of course, considered necessary and desirable by those who believe that psychologists use that autonomy in a self-serving manner to maintain patients in protracted and unnecessary treatment and/or to administer unwarranted psychological tests. The erosion of professional autonomy is, however, detrimental to the establishment and maintenance of the core relationship between professional and client. These changes in structure have also resulted in alterations of the functions of psychologists.

Functions

Traditionally, psychologists in clinical settings had three major functions: direct treatment, psychodiagnosis, and research. Direct treatment has become very goal oriented: there is an emphasis on brief interventions with people in the midst of acute episodes, with the goal of returning these individuals to adequate functioning. A number of review devices have rendered almost meaningless the "mandated mental health benefits" as legislated in many states and have forced treatment toward acute care regardless of the patient's needs as assessed by the psychologist. Group treatment has been identified as a means of addressing the problem of a shrinking amount of money available for mental health services.

Psychodiagnosis has been affected by two measures of control: 1) exclusion from benefits coverage of certain testing (such as educational evaluations) unless there is a strong indication of an Axis I diagnosis and 2) precertification of need based on a treating clinician's report. The most commonly accepted diagnostic problem is differential diagnosis of neurological impairment in children and adults through the use of neuropsychological techniques. One great area of underutilization is measurement of the degree of impairment and the degree of improvement through any of the myriad of new psychological tests. In addition, staff psychologists may be expected to generate revenue for the managed care company by providing, on a fee-for-service basis, tests and measurements that have been declared noncovered services by the company. Finally, there has been little or no emphasis on the use of either process or outcome psychotherapy research to guide the provision of services under managed care. In the early period of professional self-monitoring, this research was utilized to develop and support shorter-term treatment methods. Now the issue of refinement has become largely a fiscal one, and there is more emphasis on the technology of information management than on the realm of psychotherapy and/or psychodiagnosis.

All of these changes have impacted the daily experience of psychological practice. Private practitioners have fewer referrals of patients who are not in some way covered by managed care. Network providers receive somewhat lower fees for service. More people are seen, but they are seen less frequently. More time is devoted to paperwork without reimbursement. Employee psychologists have to move into the management track to improve their financial situations and/or to avoid very high patient contact expectations. There is some question as to whether or not psychology can maintain market share and income levels without sacrificing even more professional autonomy in this period of extensive managed care.

It would be easy to blame all of the inadequacies of mental health delivery in this country on managed care. Such a simplistic response, however, would be neither accurate nor productive. Instead of casting blame, we must look for opportunities to change the system in a meaningful way. To some extent, the scenario described above has resulted from professional psychologists' movement toward reliance on providing psychotherapy as our exclusive professional function and an inordinate emphasis on achieving parity with psychiatry at the expense of alienation from scientific psychology. We have not sufficiently diversified and evolved our roles to exploit the strengths of our profession and to ensure us of a leadership status in the provision of mental health services in this country. If we wish to safeguard our role as psychotherapists, we need to be functioning simultaneously in all of the realms that define the practice of psychology. If we do not, we risk a decline in the status and autonomy of our profession.

The PRACTICE Acronym Model

The PRACTICE Acronym Model provides a blueprint from which every psychologist can build a comprehensive practice. The eight components of the acronym can be individually blended to suit the tastes of diverse psychologists. Resultant practices should be sufficiently robust to endure transient changes in health care. We must apply our training and experience in ways that will enable us to be more than clinical technicians. If we do not continue to evolve in our roles, these roles will be defined for us by external forces such as managed care. As major health care reform becomes imminent, we cannot afford to let that happen.

What follows is a model for psychological practice that can guide us as we grapple with managed care. One highly effective way to counteract the negative impact of managed care is to structure psychological practices in such ways as to highlight and harness the unique combination of strengths that constitute our profession.

PRACTICE is an acronym that stands for the following elements:

P sychotherapy and assessment
R esearch
A ssociation and political involvement
C ommunity service
T eaching
I nterdisciplinary collaboration
C ontinuing education
E thical practice

Space constraints preclude a detailed accounting of each component of the PRACTICE Acronym Model. Instead, we highlight one aspect of each component or dimension of practice that could assist any practicing psychologist in becoming better prepared to respond to the challenges of managed care in particular and of health care reform in general.

Psychotherapy and Assessment

To the extent that our psychotherapeutic interventions are based on the ongoing assessment of patient needs, the psychologist has a defendable basis for any treatment recommendations that are made. For that reason, we must strive to specify clearly the conditions for which treatment is sought and to make informed clinical interventions guided by some theoretical understanding of psychological functioning and change. And as the profession involved in psychological testing, we must find new ways to demonstrate the cost-effectiveness of this valuable psychotherapeutic tool.

Research

The training of most psychologists in the scientist-practitioner tradition should enable us to bring some level of systematic inquiry to our work. Research is far more than formal outcome studies. If our clinical work is guided by both formal research findings and ongoing hypothesis testing, then we again put ourselves in a position where we can justify our treatment decisions to those who might challenge us.

Association and Political Involvement

Like it or not, we live in a world in which skillful systematic integration of assessment, treatment, and outcome in our psychotherapeutic work may not be enough. We may have to do more if we want to reach those in positions to control the outcome of the health care debate. We must find ways to ensure access to psychological health services during this time when restricted access and no access at all are far too common. Our state and provincial associations, working along with the American Psychological Association, have made tremendous inroads toward convincing legislators of the essential need for access to high-quality mental health services. In this regard, several state psychological associations have been instrumental in getting legislation passed that regulates managed care practices. As full-scale health care reform becomes more of a reality, we must be positioned to advocate strongly for inclusion of a rational mental health benefit.

Community Service

Our clinical work and political advocacy will ring hollow if we neglect those segments of society that remain at risk for being completely neglected by mental health care delivery systems. We must each ask ourselves whether we are contributing sufficiently to the public interest through pro bono work and community service. The major pro bono initiatives (e.g., Head Start, disaster relief network) undertaken by the Practice Directorate of the American Psychological Association have already demonstrated that by giving we distinguish ourselves as a profession.

Teaching

In the debates about the proper role for psychologists, the teaching function is often overlooked. But the fact of the matter is that psychologists have a deep-rooted tradition as teachers. We must apply that heritage to our clinical practices so that we are looked upon by managed care as the profession to train and supervise other professionals. In medical schools and undergraduate lecture halls and at conventions and in our consulting rooms, we must develop our skills as teachers and supervisors as a way of fortifying our professional roles.

Interdisciplinary Collaboration

At the same time that we distinguish ourselves, we will best serve the public's health care needs if we are seen as an integral part of any health care delivery system. Therefore, we must continue the uphill climb for recognition in the medical community. This recognition will only happen if we find new ways to collaborate on an interdisciplinary basis to bring psychological health services into the mainstream of health care. We have made major inroads through health psychology, behavioral medicine, and medical psychology, as well as through the extensive body of literature demonstrating that medical costs are reduced by use of psychological services. We owe it to the public to promote interdisciplinary collaboration in such a way as to increase the likelihood that other professionals will recognize and utilize psychological health services. And of course, our ethical principles require that we confer in an interdisciplinary manner when problems lie outside our area of competence.

Continuing Education

The importance of continuing education to our professional identity cannot be overstated. Not only do we have an ethical responsibility to remain current on the literature and apprised of new treatment developments, but we also have a commitment to do so as part of our scientist-practitioner heritage. We should strive to be thought of as the continuing-education profession.

Ethical Practice

As psychologists, we can be proud of our commitment to ethical standards of conduct. The "Ethical Principles of Psychologists" (American Psychological Association 1992) are looked to by other professions as a basis for their ethical guidelines. These principles course through the veins of our profession and as such are easily applicable to all of the components of the PRACTICE Acronym Model. From our roles as teachers and researchers to our trusted positions behind the closed doors of our offices, we must be guided at every turn by these ethical principles.

Managed care is raising many new ethical challenges. We will look to the ethics of our discipline for guidance in navigating the murky waters in which we find ourselves. Our ethical principles can serve as the beacon for all of mental health care during this period of turbulence and change.

Conclusion

Integration of the components of the PRACTICE Acronym Model is not a simple matter. We must struggle to develop contexts in which such integration is possible. We have a responsibility to ourselves, our profession, and the public good to do so.

Many psychologists have been unhappy about the changes brought about by managed care. We have seen our autonomy eroded and the public's access to psychological services seriously curtailed. At this time of skyrocketing health care costs, that presents a shameful paradox. As psychologists, we know very well that access to high-quality, cost-effective mental health services reduces the need for costly psychiatric hospitalizations. Furthermore, the costs of such services are more than offset by a reduction in utilization of medical services.

Where managed care companies act reasonably to combine cost concerns with responsible clinical practices, we must be prepared to work with them. But we must also evolve our practices so that we can assume leadership roles in the provision of mental health services in this country. If rationing and lowered professional incomes are the future, we must address this reality with a maximum of professional integrity firmly anchored in the science of psychology. Only our professional autonomy and livelihoods hang in the balance. Only the public's access to needed mental health care is at stake.

Recommended Reading

Abrahamson DJ: A scientist-practitioner organization responds to the challenges of managed mental health care. Psychotherapy in Private Practice 11:21–27, 1992

Abrahamson DJ: Managed care and psychological P.R.A.C.T.I.C.E.: an acronym for our future. Paper presented at the annual meeting of the American Psychological Association, Washington, DC, August 1992

Abrahamson DJ, Pearlman LA: The need for scientist-practitioner employ-
ment settings. Am Psychol 48:59–60, 1993

American Psychological Association: Ethical principles of psychologists
and code of conduct. Am Psychol 47:1597–1611, 1992

Lucco AA, Schreter RK: Fiscal versus clinical management of mental
health services. Paper presented at the annual midwinter meeting of Di-
visions 29 and 42, American Psychological Association, Palm Springs,
California, March 1990

The Role of the Social Worker

The Managed Care View

NORMAN WINEGAR, A.C.S.W., L.C.S.W.[*]

The advent of managed mental health care as the dominant private-sector delivery system for clinical services has provided numerous new opportunities for social workers. Managed care is a dynamic force that promises to continue shaping social work practice in the foreseeable future. Tracing its origins to both public and private settings, the social work profession has always emphasized core practice skills that resonate with present-day managed care philosophies.

Early social work practitioners and writers espoused the theme that social work—uniquely among the helping professions—viewed the presenting client, family, or group as a product of social relationships. The view recognized that biological, cultural, economic, and social relationships impacted individual behavior. This early focus on the person-envi-

---

[*]Executive Director of MCC Behavioral Care, Richmond, Virginia; clinical administrator in managed care settings.

ronment interaction helped distinguish and differentiate social workers from other helping professions (Hamilton 1951). Early on, social work case managers assessed the needs of their clients with this holistic paradigm of how various, complex factors influence human behavior. They developed, implemented, and monitored individualized treatment plans based on such assessments.

This approach to practice lends itself well to work in today's managed care environment with its "biopsychosocial assessments," "care managers," and focus on treatment services provided in the most natural setting appropriate to each client.

In addition to an approach to client services that is complementary to managed care, social workers have long confronted a challenge brought to the forefront today by managed care systems: the dilemma of serving dual clients—the individual client (or patient) and the organizational client (the employer, health maintenance organization [HMO], or other payer of services). Early in this century, a majority of large employers utilized occupational social workers to assist their employees in resolving personal, economic, social, and cultural problems at a time when the work force was becoming increasingly urban, multiethnic, and feminine (Popple 1981).

These employer-sponsored counseling services eventually dwindled and disappeared only to reemerge in the 1960s and 1970s in the form of employee assistance programs (EAPs). These assessment and referral services were instituted by employers in an effort to reduce the negative effects on their work forces of alcoholism, drug abuse, and emotional, family, and other problems. The EAP field has historically been heavily represented by professionally trained social workers accustomed to balancing the individual client's needs for appropriate services and the employer's interest in maintaining a healthy, productive work force. Such a tradition has well prepared the social work profession for service in a managed care environment—an environment in which social workers must not only advocate for clients' treatment needs but also function as a partner with employer-sponsored delivery systems focused on cost-effectiveness, efficiency, and accountability for how valuable health care resources are utilized.

Emerging managed care delivery systems have provided access for new consumer groups to the services of clinical social workers. Most managed care entities have been quick to embrace the social work profession as a key source of providers in their networks established to serve the mental health and substance abuse treatment needs of HMO members or employee populations. Before the introduction of such systems, many traditional indemnity insurance plans provided benefit coverage only for the services of psychiatrists and psychologists. Managed care systems, cognizant that social workers are cost-effective providers of care, have incorporated social workers into their networks. For example, MCC Behavioral Care, a Minneapolis-based managed care company founded by a social worker in 1974, maintains a nationwide network of mental health care providers, over 30% of whom are clinical social workers.

Managed care's gatekeeping function has helped facilitate this access to social work services. For example, in managed care systems, consumers are directed toward the appropriate type, intensity, and setting of care, as well as toward the most appropriate provider of care. If an episode of family therapy can be provided equally well by a clinical social worker and by a provider whose services are more expensive, the consumer will likely be referred to the clinical social worker. The social worker's cost-effective interventions serve not only the client's treatment goals but also the overall system's goals of efficiency and cost containment. Through such strategies, managed care systems seek to ensure that resources are available to clients who have extensive treatment needs.

Given the wide variation in practice patterns, not all social work practitioners may be successful providers in managed care systems.

Characteristics of clinical social workers often associated with a successful partnership with managed care systems in the delivery of services to clients include the following:

- ✢ An orientation toward outpatient therapy services
- ✢ Familiarity with and skill in problem-focused treatment interventions
- ✢ Awareness of the contributions of other treatment professionals and the multidisciplinary team approach, because managed care providers must sometimes refer clients to other settings as clinical needs change
- ✢ Effective practice management, thereby reducing costs and increasing the efficiency of services delivered
- ✢ A willingness to participate in the processes of increased accountability associated with managed care systems

One of the key roles performed by clinical social workers in managed care systems is that of the case manager or care manager. This clinician provides the interface between the client, the care provider, and the variety of other resources available to assist in the treatment planning process and in implementation of treatment services. Social workers in these frontline positions help managed care systems carry out their mission of ensuring that patients have access to needed services in the most appropriate setting. Clinical acumen, a knowledge of treatment and community resources, and an ability to take a collegial, collaborative approach to interactions with providers of care are essential for these professionals.

The following case example helps to clarify both the role of the social worker as care manager and the clinical processes within a managed mental health care system:

Mrs. F.'s EAP counselor called the care manager saying that Mrs.F. was at her office in a crisis state and was in need of further assessment and care. Mrs. F. was a 45-year-old married mother of two teenagers who had come to see the EAP counselor at the suggestion of a co-worker at her manufacturing plant. She had told the counselor of her increasing unhappiness, sadness, depression, and marital problems. She had expressed suicidal ideations and the thought that her family would be better off without her. The care manager spoke directly with the client and, with her approval, arranged for further evaluation despite the lateness in the business day of the call.

Mrs. F. was referred to a hospital-based, nonadmission crisis intervention program where she could be assessed while in a safe environment. The care manager spoke with the psychiatrist who evaluated Mrs. F.'s condition. In consultation with the managed care system's consulting psychiatrist and in accordance with the firm's practice guide (which had been previously shared with the treating psychiatrist), it was recommended to Mrs. F. that she be admitted to inpatient care for further stabilization. The care manager coordinated these services with her family, the EAP professional, and her primary care physician. The care manager also authorized health care benefit coverage, both for the professional services and for the services at the managed care system–affiliated facility.

During Mrs. F.'s 4-day hospital stay, the care manager was in close contact with the hospital's nonphysician staff, as well as the attending psychiatrist, concerning discharge planning. Using the managed care firm's practice guides and in consultation with the firm's consulting psychiatrist, the care manager and the attending psychiatrist agreed that Mrs. F. was ready for discharge to a less-intensive level of care based on Mrs. F.'s progress and symptoms. The care manager arranged an appointment for Mrs. F. on the day of discharge with a social worker who offered an intensive treatment program appropriate to Mrs. F.'s treatment needs. Benefit coverage for Mrs. F.'s continuing care at the psychiatrist's office was also arranged.

After 2 weeks of daily treatment, Mrs. F. had improved enough to return to her job, and her contacts with the social worker were reduced to a weekly and then a monthly basis. Eventually, the social worker–provider and the social worker–care manager agreed that Mrs. F. no longer required therapy contacts and the treatment was discontinued, although she continued to receive treatment from the psychiatrist for several months more. At that time, she was returned to the care of her primary care physician who, in consultation with the psychiatrist, monitored and ultimately discontinued her medications because of her recovery.

Throughout this treatment episode, the care manager periodically reviewed Mrs. F.'s progress with the treatment provider, more intensively at first and then less frequently as Mrs. F. progressed. The care manager coordinated all the services among the various mental health professionals, as well as among the other professionals involved in the case. Benefit coverage was preauthorized by the care manager at appropriate points throughout this episode of care, assuring the treating professionals and facilities that they would be compensated for their services (excepting mandatory client copayments). Both the managed care staff and the treatment providers utilized a practice guide that helped them to direct the client to the most appropriate level and intensity of care within the managed care's network continuum of services, as well as within its interface with primary health care systems.

In addition to providing clinical services and being care managers, social workers may also be EAP counselors in the same managed care systems. These social workers function as gatekeepers: they are the mandatory access point to the system of care, providing assessment, brief counseling, and referral to additional treatment services when appropriate. Although this function parallels the traditional role of an EAP counselor, requiring that mental health services be accessed through the EAP gatekeeper and integrating the EAP function with the managed care network are recent innovations.

Opportunities for social workers in managed care systems do not end with these roles but include jobs in administrative areas. These jobs can be broadly classified into three groups: network management, account management, and operations management.

Social work administrators in managed mental health care systems provide important network management functions. These include recruiting, screening, and orienting new providers. In addition to screening for appropriate credentials such as licensure, network managers attempt to select providers whose treatment philosophy and practice patterns are most closely aligned with the practice guidelines endorsed by the managed care firm. Network managers also evaluate affiliated providers' practice patterns and conduct quality assurance activities in an effort to upgrade the standard of care delivered by the network as a whole. Such network management activities may also include contracting with inpatient facilities, negotiation of hospital bed per diems, and various other related activities.

Account management activities provided by social work administrators include presale technical support to sales and marketing staff, reporting of utilization data to customers, and ongoing customer relations activities. The opportunity to assist customer companies' benefits administrators in designing mental health and substance abuse treatment benefits can be an especially rewarding experience for clinical social work administrators.

Some social workers employed in the administration of managed care systems not only manage networks of providers and fulfill account management activities but also manage clinical offices. These operations employ practitioners to provide direct services to clients. Staff recruitment, supervision, and evaluation—as well as program development, financial planning, and management—are some of the responsibilities these administrators share. Other duties include oversight of provider claims payment, customer (client) service functions, and quality management activities.

As managed mental health care systems proliferate, many new opportunities will be available to social work clinicians, particularly to those who can blend the clinical, managerial, and organizational skills necessary to develop services for this growing market. For some social workers, this will mean applying previously learned skills to a new context. For others, it will mean retooling, becoming adept at new treatment approaches or practice in new settings.

Emerging managed care systems present challenges and opportunities for social work educators as well. Social work education at both the university and the continuing professional education levels must be modified to give necessary attention to these evolving delivery systems and the rapidly expanding array of innovative services being developed to meet the needs of clients. Social work educators and managed care clinicians must develop meaningful administrative and clinical practicum experiences for graduate students. Professional associations such as the National Association of Social Workers and others should explore jointly sponsored training and educational activities with universities and the managed care industry. These efforts will better prepare the profession for effective partnerships with the payer community aimed at enhancing services to clients in the years to come.

References

Hamilton G: Theory and Practice of Social Case Work, 2nd Edition. New York, Columbia University Press, 1951

Popple PR: Social work practice in business and industry 1875–1930. Social Service Review 55(2):257–269, 1981

Recommended Reading

Strategies and Solutions: The Journal of Managed Mental Health Care. Bloomington, MN, Strategies and Solutions Press

Straussner SLA (ed): Occupational Social Work Today. New York, Haworth, 1989

Winegar N: The Clinician's Guide to Managed Mental Health Care. New York, Haworth, 1992

Winegar N, Bistline JL: Marketing Mental Health Services to Managed Care. New York, Haworth, 1994

The Clinician's View

MARY JO MONAHAN, L.C.S.W.*

The majority of clinical social workers in the United States work in health- and mental health–related fields in both the public and private sectors. From Social Security in the 1930s to Medicare/Medicaid and the Community Mental Health Act in the 1960s, publicly subsidized programs had been the primary "environmental context" in which clinical social workers worked. As a result, social workers traditionally were associated with the poor, the disadvantaged, and the oppressed.

In the 1970s and 1980s, as employers became more involved in maintaining the mental health of their workers, private counseling agencies were used to offer mental health services to employees and their families. Clinical social workers migrated into these settings as well as into the workplace. As a result, the clientele served by clinical social workers expanded to include middle- and upper-income families.

Regardless of the practice setting, income level, or cultural diversity of the clients, the unifying and primary mission of the clinical social worker always has been to enhance the individual's and family's social functioning, as well as to solve social problems. This dual focus recognizes and supports the reciprocal responsibilities of society and its members to each other and is fundamental to the clinical social worker's approach to service delivery.

Another distinguishing approach of the clinical social worker is the "person-in-environment" perspective that views clients in the context of all the systems in which they function. The clinical social worker "starts where the client is" and assesses the individual's as well as the system's strengths and weaknesses. Successful interaction with the environment

---

*Clinical social worker in private practice, associated with Psychotherapy and Employee Assistance Consultants, Tampa, Florida; Chairperson, Competence Certification Commission, National Association of Social Workers; Adjunct Professor, School of Social Work, University of South Florida, Tampa, Florida.

leads to a sense of competence and self-worth. Although the environment may provide resources and opportunities to support the client, it also may erect barriers that interfere with the client's functioning. Clinical social work interventions are designed to effect both individual and systemic change.

As providers of mental health care, clinical social workers operate in two critical roles simultaneously. We are clinicians for clients—the individual, family, or group—and are also advocates. As clinicians, we diagnose, assess, and treat the full range of psychosocial problems and challenges that clients face in the course of daily living: childbirth, school adjustments, marriage, parenting, job stress, divorce, depression, anxiety, physical and sexual abuse, addictions, long-term physical illness, chronic mental illness, financial burdens, aging, and death.

Yet the clinical social worker's ethical responsibility, professional training, and social interests extend beyond the client to encompass systemic challenges. Like all citizens, clinical social workers and their clients are profoundly affected by the social, economic, cultural, and political context in which they live. Clinical social workers advocate for necessary change within these contexts to ensure adequate and comprehensive service delivery that is nondiscriminatory and accessible to those in need.

In the 1990s, managed mental health care companies are emerging as the new environmental context for the delivery of mental health services. Employers who bear the skyrocketing cost of mental health and substance abuse treatment through indemnity insurance plans have been the impetus for this change. The stated goal of most managed mental health care companies is to increase access to quality treatment for clients while maintaining cost-effective utilization of mental health and substance abuse benefits for the payers. The payer's dual responsibility both to provide treatment to the client and to maintain cost savings for the system parallels the dual-role challenge of the clinical social worker within the managed care environment.

I believe that because of our training, experience, history, and perspective, we clinical social workers are comfortable with our dual roles as clinician and advocate. Most of us, at some time in our careers, have been employed in agency settings such as child welfare, public or private schools and hospitals, or home health care. Agency policies and practices often pose ethical dilemmas and treatment paradoxes for both the clinician and the employing agency. Social workers accept the responsibility for improving the functioning of the system as well as the functioning of individuals.

In the remainder of this section, I highlight some specific elements of managed mental health care that need to be improved.

Managed care presents a three-way relationship. There are a client, a clinician, and a payer, all interconnected (Figure 9–1). As clinicians, we view triangles as a common and natural process for couples struggling to adapt to their roles as new parents or as a disruptive process when one spouse is having an extramarital affair or is addicted. Disruptive triangles are based on competition, tight control over limited resources, and a style of either/or problem solving that is ineffective and carries long-term negative consequences for all participants. No one is happy, nor is anyone getting his or her needs met, and the tension continues to mount.

The clinical intervention is to help all participants understand the

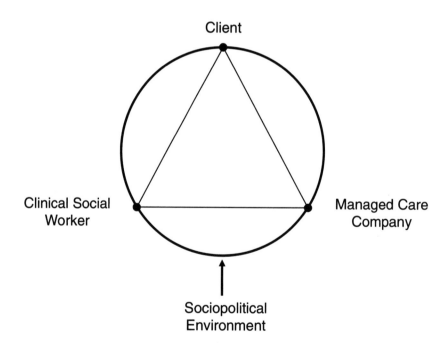

Figure 9–1. The managed care triangle: a three-way relationship among client, clinical social worker, and managed care company.

impact of one relationship on the others, as well as the choices and responsibilities of each participant. The clinical goal is to move to a cooperation-based triangle where the tension in the relationship is used to creatively benefit the whole. Obligation and accountability flow among all participants, as do need and choice.

The application of this problem-solving style to the triangle of relationships among the client, clinician, and payer could be very effective and could lead to long-term benefits. Because the primary goal of both the clinician and the payer is service to the client, cooperation, rather than competition, encourages mutually created solutions.

With managed care, client confidentiality is a problem. Collaboration between the client and the clinician is based on trust and caring. Trust is based, in part, on the confidential nature of the communication between clinician and client. Yet the payer requires sufficient information to determine the appropriate level of care and length of treatment and to ensure accountability and cost-effectiveness. Clinical social workers are often caught in the middle between providing a confidential atmosphere for the client while providing enough information to the gatekeepers for the payer to authorize ongoing treatment.

In addition, the clinical social worker has no control over who has access to confidential information once it is released to the payer. Frequent turnover of case managers and the use of electronic communications can further lead to the erosion of confidentiality and may compromise trust in the helping relationship.

Clients do care about confidentiality. Here is an example:

A woman who worked for a large company sought counseling through her employee assistance program as she came to terms with the ending of her 20-year marriage and began a divorce process that was fraught with mistrust and manipulation. She was referred to a clinical social worker in private practice in the community. After a few sessions, she came in very angry and stated that a male co-worker who had been emotionally supportive of her had been advised to spend less time with her on breaks and at lunch "because it did not look good." Her initial response was to ask the clinician whether she had informed her employer about this relationship. The clinician stated that she indeed had not, and explored with the client the issues of trust that were now arising in many aspects of her life.

Clients need to be informed by the managed care company, before referral, what specific information is to be shared with whom, and for what purposes. The client's consent should be obtained before releasing information. The clinician should only record and release information that is related to treatment goals and problem resolution.

In addition, managed care companies need to develop guidelines regarding utilization of client information for purposes of research. Clinical social workers trained in clinical research can be valuable resources in establishing these guidelines.

A second area of ethical concern for clinical social workers is whether managed care provides mental health care that is sufficiently comprehensive and continuous to meet the client's needs. Clinicians are handcuffed by payers who limit conditions that will be covered for treatment or who restrict treatment modalities. Providing only crisis intervention when short-term counseling, supportive maintenance, or preventive services are indicated puts clinicians in a serious bind. The following two vignettes illustrate these points.

A 29-year-old Afro-American woman was referred through her employer. She worked in the human resources department. She presented as depressed, anxious, and exhausted. The psychosocial assessment revealed that she had been married for 3 years, her husband was employed as a paramedic, and their first daughter was 6 months old. She and her husband each were experiencing severe job, financial, and relationship stress. Their arguing had escalated into one incident of pushing and shoving that had distressed them greatly.

The clinical social worker recommended marital sessions for short-term treatment of 3–6 months' duration to focus on crisis intervention, problem solving and conflict resolution, understanding the expansion of their family roles to include parenting, and stress reduction for each partner. Instead, the managed care company authorized three sessions. Then, only two additional sessions were authorized in response to both the clients' and the clinician's requests. Because the employee's contract did not provide for coverage of marital counseling, the only option offered was to diagnose the woman with major depression and refer her to a psychiatrist. The clinician continued sessions with the couple at a further-reduced rate (the initial managed care fee was 25% less than the clinician's regular fee) rather than change the diagnosis or interrupt treatment. Although their relationship stress decreased significantly, their financial stress increased. The clinician took a major cut in pay also.

The second example illustrates how the original complaint is not always the cause of the client's distress. What looks like a problem with a brief solution can be something very different.

> A 33-year-old woman, whose daughter had just turned 6 years old, presented with complaints of poor communication, obsessive concern, and excessive anger at and criticism of her own mother. This situation was creating tension because her mother took care of her daughter while she was at work. She was preapproved for five individual sessions by the payer. During the third session, the client revealed that she had been sexually abused by a family member when she was 6 years old, and she had been experiencing flashbacks that were unnerving. When the clinician contacted the company and requested further sessions to deal with the newly uncovered crisis, she was told to deal only with the original complaint.

The clinical social worker is further challenged by clients who present with chronic conditions (e.g., addictions or personality disorders) that necessitate a longer-term treatment approach. Other situations may also require longer-term approaches. For instance, in Florida, nurses who are impaired due to drug or alcohol addiction are referred to the Intervention Project for Nurses. This project provides an alternative to disciplinary action against their professional license. As a condition of compliance, the recovering nurse may be referred for ongoing therapy. If accommodations for longer-term therapy are not available through the payers, the financial burden on clients to pay their therapy expenses out of pocket may become a barrier to their recovery process.

Simply stated, clinical social workers advocate that limiting access to preventive or appropriate mental health or substance abuse care should not become the preferred method of cost containment in the managed care environment.

For social workers, a third problem area is cultural, ethnic, and gender sensitivity in the provision of mental health care. Are the clinicians and the managed care companies adequately prepared to deal with the diversity of the clients we serve? Does the mix of clinicians match the mix of clients with respect to race, ethnic background, and gender? And are services offered where people live, or must they travel long distances to get care? Distance alone can be viewed as a discriminatory barrier against certain groups.

Another problem with managed care is that some companies incorporate a "hold harmless" clause into the contract between the payer and the clinician. Normally, an employer shares the liability for the conduct of any employee, and the employee is not held responsible for the actions of the employer. In the managed care arena, we must work toward an equitable sharing of liability and risk.

Clinical social workers have made enormous strides in acquiring professional recognition and respect from other providers of mental health services, such as psychiatrists and psychologists. However, when providing similar psychotherapeutic and counseling services, clinical social workers are often reimbursed at a lower rate than these other providers or are restricted from participating as providers. If companies feel the need for reimbursement differentials among providers of the same services, a more equitable criterion might be years of experience rather than academic degree.

Lastly, the rapid proliferation of managed care companies is itself a problem. Each company has a different corporate structure, mission, policies, and reimbursement strategies. For each case, clinicians must engage in two levels of administration, management, and documentation of services because they have two clients—the client being treated and the client who pays for the services. Clinicians are not being reimbursed for the time spent doing extra reporting and documentation. For example, clinical social workers are paid between $45 and $60 per session by managed care companies, a 20%–50% reduction over their regular fees. The added administrative and management work for each case increases the time involved by 20%, which results in a further fee reduction. These reduced fees are discouraging many experienced clinicians from entering the managed care environment. The entire system suffers the loss of our expertise.

Managed mental health care is here to stay, and clinical social workers are essential to its successful existence. Clinical social workers must contribute in three specific ways. First, we must clearly articulate and maintain their unique approach to mental health care. Second, we must develop allies within managed care systems to ensure quality clinical services to clients. Finally, we must continue to advocate for comprehensive mental health and substance abuse services for all citizens.

Section IV

Emerging Clinical Issues

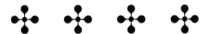

✣ 10 ✣

Practice Guidelines

The Managed Care View

JOHN BARTLETT, M.D., M.P.H.[*]

No other area of clinical practice over the last 5 years has been the subject of more debate and concern than the topic of practice guidelines. The discussions to date have involved a wide variety of interested parties, with multiple agendas and points of view. On the one hand, professional bodies, including many specialty organizations such as the American Psychiatric Association, have come to see practice guidelines as valuable educational and heuristic tools. Policymakers, on the other hand, have come to see them as a potentially powerful tool for use in cost containment and health care reform. In turn, a variety of payers, including most managed care companies, have used some form of documented standards of care, especially so-called level-of-care criteria, as tools (or weapons, depending on your point of view) in the review and management of individual cases. For the practitioner, who remains charged with the demanding task of providing care to real people whose problems and cir-

[*]Vice President and Corporate Medical Director, MCC Behavioral Care, Eden Prairie, Minnesota.

cumstances are unique and immediate, the whole subject of practice guidelines has most often produced a feeling of deep concern and a sense that such guidelines are impractical.

I know, because those were the very feelings I experienced when I was introduced to the concept of practice guidelines. At that time, in January 1989, I was only 6 months into my tenure as the corporate medical director of a managed behavioral care firm, MCC Companies (now MCC Behavioral Care). The occasion was a one-on-one meeting between myself and my new boss, a businessman who had trained as an engineer and who had for most of his career been involved in the development and operation of large management information systems.

What I came to understand over time was that it was this very background, with its strong process and systems improvement orientation, that caused my boss to see variability in any process as inherently problematic—not necessarily bad or negligent, but intrinsically wasteful, inefficient, and confusing. In the last few years, I have come to understand that many large, successful manufacturing and service organizations in this country also see process variation as a major threat to the quality of the product or service produced by that process. This realization is particularly important because these are the very organizations that have traditionally provided relatively rich mental health and substance abuse benefits to their employees. Now, these organizations are increasingly turning to so-called managed approaches in their search for an appropriate balance between cost and quality in this area of their employee benefits programs. As they do so, they often bring their management bias against process variation to an evaluation of these approaches.

In fact, like many other managers within this type of organization, my boss had reacted strongly to the wide and often unexplained variability in clinical approaches and processes he saw being used in mental health and substance abuse treatments. Furthermore, he quickly appreciated that the variability he was witnessing was not the normal variation (that which falls within acceptable limits) that any process, natural or manmade, inevitably generates. Instead, he realized he was witnessing the wide swings and fluctuations associated with ill-defined and poorly understood and managed processes. In short, he saw that he was involved in the management of processes—in this case the delivery of mental health and substance abuse services—for which no standards existed.

This lack of standards, in turn, posed a set of serious strategic challenges for my boss. To begin with, this variability and the associated difficulties in defining and documenting quality tempted many payers to limit their risk by markedly restricting available benefits. Without standards, how could he tell whether his organization was doing a good job? More importantly, how could his customers tell? In addition, without standards as the centerpiece of a responsible and responsive management process, how could he detect unacceptable variation and therefore identify opportunities for improvement?

These types of concerns led to our discussion in early 1989 during which he informed me that a major and immediate challenge for me as MCC's medical director would be the development of documented clinical standards for the organization. And it was this challenge in turn that, quite honestly, led to that sinking feeling in the pit of my stomach that many clinicians feel at the mere mention of clinical standards and practice guidelines. My immediate reaction was one of panic and confusion. I quickly thought, "He can't know what he's asking; he's an engineer and a businessman, not a clinician. You really can't do that in mental health and substance abuse care . . . they're more art than science . . . " and so on.

It is now 5 years later and MCC has just published the second edition of its practice guidelines, the *Preferred Practices,* which cover the outpatient treatment of a variety of Axis I disorders. In addition, we have a full and comprehensive set of level-of-care guidelines. Most importantly, both of these documented sets of clinical standards are used daily within the organization as part of an ongoing and continuous effort to define, monitor, and ultimately improve the care that we either provide or manage. As an organization we no longer fear the whole concept of documented standards of care; instead, we are actively involved in exploring and increasing their value in the delivery and management of clinical care.

How did we get from those immediate feelings of fear and foreboding to the level of acceptance and even reliance we now see within the organization? The key to the transition has been an increased understanding of and willingness to accept the central role of standards in the monitoring and improvement of the process of delivering care to patients.

Our quality efforts as an organization have moved over the last 5 years from traditional inspection-based approaches, which attempt to improve quality by identifying and weeding out outliers or "bad apples," to ongoing and continuous efforts to define and document what our performance should be in any given area and then to monitor and manage variation from that expected level of performance. Under this approach, the organizational process becomes one of developing standards with appropriate input from all involved parties and then attempting to understand and minimize variation from these standards. Ultimately, the theoretical role of standards changes from one that defines a standard as a threshold ("everything above is OK") to one that defines standards as ideals that have a legitimate claim to be the measure against which all else is evaluated. Therefore, the concept of "meeting" standards becomes an outmoded idea and is replaced by the concept of "molding" them.

But what does all this theory have to do with that feeling of dread and foreboding that I was left with after my conversation with my boss? After all, I was hardly convinced that the idea of developing and documenting clinical standards was achievable, never mind wise. Yet I had few, if any, choices in the matter, because I still had to report to him on a regular basis about my progress. My first thought was to look to various professional organizations for guidance, because in other fields of health care it had been these groups that had most often driven the development and dissemination of practice standards. What I found in 1989, however, was that not only had no standards or guidelines been developed in mental health and substance abuse, but also in at least some of the major professional groups there seemed to be considerable internal debate about the advisability of the very effort. In retrospect, of course, this finding made obvious sense because it merely reflected the variation in treatment approaches that had driven the need in the first place.

Therefore, I sought the support and guidance of a small group of senior clinicians within MCC. As a group we began to discuss how we might go about the process of developing and documenting practice guidelines ourselves. Fortunately, within the organization there were extensive clinical resources on which to draw. In January 1989, for example, we employed over 250 clinicians, including 50 psychiatrists, in about 20 cities; today, some 5 years later, we employ over 600 clinicians in 65 sites and contract with over 10,000 additional clinicians in over 125 cities nationally.

Much to my surprise, as I spoke with this carefully selected group of clinical opinion leaders, I found that the idea of documented clinical standards met with uniform approval and even excitement! The general reaction was, in fact, overwhelmingly positive. Buoyed by this finding, I myself became excited by the challenge. As a first step, I decided to find out more about what the average (if there is such an animal) clinician thought about the concept of practice guidelines. Therefore, I hired a group who specialized in performing health care–oriented market research to explore the level of understanding and comfort of clinicians (including a sampling of those in private practice) with the concept of clinical standards.

Before I describe what we found from this exercise, let me digress for just a moment to explain what we at MCC mean when we speak of practice guidelines. The key to understanding their role and functions for us lies in the definition of the word "guide." *Webster's Ninth New Collegiate Dictionary* defines a guide as "a device for steadying the motion or direction of something." Therefore, the central concept is one of *directing,* not controlling. In fact, we see practice guidelines as a tool for managing variability in clinical practice by informing the clinical judgment of clinicians. The guidelines do so by addressing that aspect of clinical judgment that one noted author, Dr. Alvan Feinstein of Yale, has called the therapeutic component—that which addresses the question "What is the best treatment for this disorder?" In so doing, we distinguish guidelines from protocols, which we see as being far more restrictive and directive. Protocols are best considered as promoting strict adherence to a "correct" procedure and therefore as restricting discussion rather than fostering it. To our way of thinking, protocols are best seen as a tool for the limited delegation of authority under strictly defined conditions, as in the protocols nurses or physician assistants routinely use in the ambulatory detoxification of patients.

Using these principles to structure their efforts, the market researchers over the next month or so contacted a number of clinicians in 11 regions of the country. These interviews revealed a number of interesting findings. To begin with, although many clinicians were initially wary of the concept, almost all ultimately accepted and even supported the use of clinical standards. In addition, most were able to identify potential applications for them that the clinicians themselves found useful. These applications included use of the clinical standards as a tool for self-assessment, for promoting discussion among peers, and, finally, for focused training and education. Interestingly enough, many clinicians voiced the opinion that an important function of standards was to protect patients by fostering state-of-the-art approaches to treatment. On the negative side, the providers uniformly expressed concern that any set of standards be developed by practicing clinicians, not by academics or researchers and certainly not by business people.

With this information in mind, we formed a number of teams, each charged with looking at a different major diagnostic cluster within the American Psychiatric Association's *Diagnostic and Statistical Manual of Mental Disorders, 3rd Edition, Revised.* Each team was headed by one of the senior clinicians identified earlier and was composed of 8–12 providers with identified expertise (e.g., publications, university appointments) in the identified clinical area. Each team, using standardized computer-based searches, reviewed the available professional literature and developed specific recommendations. These in turn were reviewed by the senior clinicians as a group for content and tone and then returned to the working groups for revision. The final document was edited and published under my direction, using specific guidance developed by the market researchers in their earlier telephone interviews with the clinicians.

This approach has served our organization well and has remained essentially unchanged throughout the development and publication of both our level-of-care guidelines in late 1990 and the second edition of the *Preferred Practices* in 1992. The major change in approach has been the increased participation of non-MCC clinicians. For the first edition, about 15 of the 75 providers involved did not work for MCC; for the second edition, more than 30 clinicians, including 4 of the 7 team leaders, were from outside the organization. In addition, over the last 5 years the American Academy of Child and Adolescent Psychiatry and the American Psychiatric Association have themselves begun publishing guidelines. As these become available, we routinely review the corresponding guidelines in the *Preferred Practices.* To date, in the areas of attention-deficit hyperactivity disorder, conduct disorder, and eating disorders, there has been general agreement between the two efforts.

As a whole, the *Preferred Practices* address seven broad classes of clinical presentations: disruptive behavior disorders, eating disorders, psychotic disorders, mood disorders, anxiety disorders, adjustment disorders, and psychoactive substance abuse disorders. Within each practice guideline are five major components. The first is a referral (or triage) decision between psychiatric and nonpsychiatric clinicians that is structured according to objective clinical criteria. Each guideline then proceeds to a broad description of what constitutes an appropriate intervention, a list of defined end points for treatment, and a set of alternative treatment strategies in case adequate progress is not being made toward the defined end points. A second, separate volume contains the theoretical and research support for the interventions contained in the guidelines themselves.

How do we use these guidelines in our efforts to define and improve the quality of the care we deliver or manage? Within our own clinical operations, they function as the basis for multidisciplinary treatment planning and case review and have served to greatly increase and standardize, among other things, clinical referrals to psychiatrists. In addition, they serve as the foundation for many of our internal training programs.

In fact, as a routine part of MCC's quality management program, each of our 65 offices nationally reviews a 1% sample of cases (or 25 cases, whichever is greater), chosen centrally and at random by our management information system, against the appropriate preferred practice. The information derived from this random case review is used both to identify opportunities to improve patient care within our offices and to improve and develop the practice guidelines themselves. An excellent example of the latter is how our practice guideline for substance abuse was changed between the first and the second editions by using feedback from the random case review.

In the first edition of the *Preferred Practices,* part of the practice guideline required each patient's substance abuse history and course to be reviewed against the Jellinek criteria. In late 1990, as we reviewed a national sample of cases against this standard, we found that only 35% had documented evidence of such a review. A traditional inspection-based approach to quality at that point would have gone something like this: "The standard has not been met; you will be reviewed again, and we had better find 80% (or 90% or whatever) compliance with the standard."

Instead, we adopted an improvement-oriented approach, which went something like this: "You folks developed the original standard; it wasn't imposed on you. Now we find that you're not following it. Why not?" The explanation was that although the Jellinek criteria were time honored and provided strong linkage to Alcoholics Anonymous and the fellowship movement, they were somewhat dated and did not address all forms of alcohol abuse (e.g., binge drinking) or other drug use (e.g., crack, prescription drugs). The feeling, therefore, was that they did not represent a sound assessment tool in many cases. There was, however, general agreement that they were a strong tool to promote motivation for treatment in patients. Therefore, in the second edition of the *Preferred Practices* the revised standard has all patients being assisted in conducting a *self-assessment* against the Jellinek criteria.

In our network-based operations, where all care is provided by contracted clinicians in their offices, we have concentrated on using the guidelines to standardize our care management process. Many clinicians in practice are appropriately concerned about the qualifications and training of the care managers with whom they interact. At MCC, we have attempted to respond positively to these concerns not just by hiring fully trained, licensed, and experienced mental health and substance abuse clinicians but also by providing these clinicians with clearly documented clinical standards to assist and inform their judgment in the review of individual cases. In so doing, we have assured our network providers that our care managers are applying clear standards that are supported by experience and research, not simply "making it up as they go along." In fact, within the National Service Center of MCC, where we perform the care management services for our employer accounts, each care manager's performance in applying the standards is monitored monthly, and areas for improvement are identified. The focus here is not on the clinicians and whether or not they follow the guidelines; instead, it is on the care managers and whether or not they do! The goal is to reduce the variation our care managers add to the treatment process, so as to better understand the differences among the providers with whom we work.

All of these activities are examples of how we at MCC have tried to use documented clinical standards as the foundation for an improvement-oriented approach to defining and monitoring the delivery of mental health and substance abuse care. To date, we have employed both process-oriented interventions (e.g., the monitoring of care managers and the random review of cases) and content-oriented ones (e.g., the revision of standards as clinical consensus changes). In all of these, a primary goal has been to minimize and better understand the variability in clinical practice and approach that has marked the delivery of mental health and substance abuse care for at least the last two or three decades.

Yet the reduction and minimization of variability clearly are not enough. Although it is true that the judicious application and use of documented clinical standards allow us to do a better job of limiting variability, are our standards correct? Are we, in fact, limiting variability around the right ideal? Standards developed by consensus, after all, at best represent a distillation of the state of knowledge at any given point in time. It has been correctly pointed out that the consensus standard about ether anesthesia before 1846 in Boston most likely would have been that this type of anesthesia was the devil's work. Within our own areas of clinical experience, we have examples such as the treatment of acute psychosis before the introduction of neuroleptics and the treatment of obsessive-compulsive disorder before clomipramine. Therefore, the strategic challenge with consensus standards is that consensus—by definition—limits variability, but it may not always reflect the truth. In fact, it can even be used to frustrate efforts to redefine and improve a process.

Fortunately, current developments in the organization and delivery of mental health and substance abuse care will soon be better able to address these legitimate concerns. To date, in my opinion, the era of managed care has gone through two generations and is on the verge of entering yet a third. The first generation, the age of utilization review, was characterized by attempts to limit variability in clinical practice through coercion and even confrontation. These early efforts represented almost a pure inspection approach to quality, with proprietary standards and no formal, agreed-on relationship between the provider and the reviewer.

The second generation, which is now widely in place throughout the country, represents the era of consent. There is increased sharing of standards and approaches and more or less careful selection of providers based on gross estimations of compatibility and "managed care–friendliness." With these network-based approaches, there are defined contractual responsibilities and duties for both parties—the managed care vendor as well as the provider.

This second generation, however, is already being replaced by a third. This new era will be marked by the development of truly organized health care delivery systems, distinguished by closely linked relationships among purchasers, managed care vendors, and carefully selected providers. These organized delivery systems will provide the infrastructure for the documentation and improvement of standards of care. Practice guidelines and critical pathways for care will be used as a part of these systems' routine operations. Most importantly, the outcomes of these applications will be measured and evaluated in methodologically sound ways with valid and reliable instruments that have been adapted and modified for use in practice environments. These outcomes will address a number of domains of interest, including areas such as clinical improvement; role functioning at work, school, and in the family or community; utilization of medical and surgical services; disability, including sick leave, absenteeism, and worker's compensation; and productivity.

If all that sounds merely high-minded and futuristic, I can assure you it is not. MCC, for example, has been working with health services researchers from the University of Minnesota for the last year in developing and implementing a scientifically sound approach to the collection and analysis of outcome data on substance abuse treatment. This approach is designed around data collection tools that are practical as well as valid and reliable. Future applications will look at mood disorders and anxiety disorders, among others.

This vision, then, would transform the normal business and clinical operations of managed care providers from a focus on inspection to a focus on improvement. It would make their normal activities supportive of the examination and empirical demonstration of the value of mental health and substance abuse treatment. Within the vision, practice guidelines developed collaboratively and applied sensitively become both the foundation for understanding and measuring the results of different approaches and the means of codifying proven ones. Therefore, when practice guidelines and outcomes evaluation are truly linked in unified, organized delivery systems, they have the potential to become major tools in the preservation and even the expansion of adequate and appropriate mental health and substance abuse benefits. To this end, they become important not just to payers, providers, and policymakers but also to our patients.

The Clinician's View

JOHN S. MCINTYRE, M.D.[*]

In the past decade, there has been an explosion in the development of practice guidelines. Initially viewed with suspicion by clinicians, guidelines that are developed by the profession are now seen as potentially very helpful in maintaining a clinical perspective as the health care system continues to evolve.

Actually, practice guidelines in various forms have existed for many years. The American Psychiatric Association has promulgated guidelines almost from its inception in 1844. In 1851, the Association (at that time called the Association of Medical Superintendents of American Institutions for the Insane) adopted 26 propositions on the construction of institutions for mentally ill persons. These propositions were very detailed and specific. In the following year, a complementary set of propositions concerning the staffing of these institutions was approved by the members of the association. Although initially labeled propositions, what we have come to call guidelines were frequently issued under the title "task force reports." For example, there was a task force report on the benzodiazepines, one on electroconvulsive therapy, and the extensive and very highly regarded *Task Force Report on Treatment of Psychiatric Disorders* edited by Dr. Byram Karasu.

In 1989 the American Psychiatric Association voted to initiate a formal practice guideline project in which guidelines for treatment of specific psychiatric disorders would be developed and approved by the membership (through the Assembly of District Branches and the Board of Trustees). The first guideline to be approved was the practice guideline for eating disorders published in the *American Journal of Psychiatry* in February 1993. The second was the practice guideline for major depres-

[*]President, American Psychiatric Association; private practice in psychiatry, Rochester, New York; Chair, Department of Psychiatry, St. Mary's Hospital, Rochester, New York; and Clinical Professor of Psychiatry, University of Rochester, Rochester, New York.

sive disorder in adults (published in April 1993 in the same journal). Guidelines on schizophrenia, bipolar disorder, addictive disorders, panic disorder, Alzheimer's disease, and the diagnostic evaluation of adults are now being developed.

Problems With Current Criteria

Although practice guidelines are developed primarily to educate professionals, many clinicians are hopeful that these guidelines will help address a number of problems that have arisen in this era of increased review and authorization of treatment plans. Clinicians discussing problems in utilization review and many managed care programs identify five common complaints about the criteria that are currently used to determine the appropriateness of clinical care:

1. Frequently the criteria are arbitrary and not based on research data or clinical consensus.
2. When the criteria are based on research data, frequently the data are out of date.
3. Generally, the criteria do not take into account the complexity of the clinical situation, including issues of comorbidity and unique features of the individual case that alter decisions about treatment alternatives.
4. The criteria are often "secret," and in discussions between a clinician and reviewer there is not a common language.
5. The case material is reviewed by professionals who do not know the patient and frequently are not at the same level of expertise or experience as the treating professional.

Despite these frequent problems, most clinicians recognize and accept that a legitimate need for increased accountability has evolved and that third-party payers and managed care companies expect that the care rendered will be the most effective for the money spent. One side of the challenge is how to review and preview care so that the third-party payer or managed care company can ascertain that the care being rendered is indeed medically necessary and cost-effective. At the same time, clinicians should insist that the review or preview be reasonable from a clinical standpoint and flexible enough to take into account individual variability and patient need. Practice guidelines, especially if they are accepted by both the practitioner and the reviewer or managed care company, can be part of the solution to these challenging issues.

Let us examine how practice guidelines can impact on the five problem areas identified above.

Arbitrary Data

Well-developed practice guidelines should be based on good research data and solid clinical consensus. With the tremendous increase in data that has emerged in the past two decades, practice guidelines can be a significant help to clinicians in placing these studies in perspective and in determining their implications for clinical decision making. Because of the voluminous number and at times contradictory nature of some of these studies, it is important to involve recognized experts in the research area being described. Further, the guidelines must make clear the methods of the literature review and describe the strengths as well as the weaknesses of the available studies. Similarly, in forming opinions about clinical consensus, clinicians with a breadth of clinical expertise and experience must be utilized and, as with research data, the source of the clinical consensus and how "solid" the consensus is should be made explicit.

Data Out of Date

Because of the rapid advances both in technology and in clinical research, guidelines should be reviewed and revised at regular intervals, not less frequently than 3- to 5-year intervals. This is the length of time proposed by both the American Psychiatric Association and the American Medical Association for reviewing and rewriting practice guidelines.

Comorbidity and Individual Variation

Clinically useful guidelines must reflect the reality that comorbidity is a frequent occurrence and, further, that other individual biological and psychosocial variables can significantly affect a patient's responsiveness to specific therapeutic initiatives. These issues—comorbidity and "special circumstances"—may result in guidelines that are lengthy, over-inclusive, and very general. For guidelines to be useful, there must be a balancing attempt to be concise and specific. Both clinician and reviewer must recognize that guidelines are strategies to be followed in a large majority of cases and that exceptions are not infrequent and fairly easy to justify. Practice parameters are categorized by a number of authors (including Dr. David Eddy) into "standards," "guidelines," and "options." Standards are more rigidly defined: the recommended action is expected to be followed in essentially all cases. Exceptions are rare and difficult to justify. At the other end of the spectrum are options, which apply to situations where there is no preferred choice of treatment. Summarizing these issues, each American Psychiatric Association guideline has a "statement of intent" that notes:

> This report is not intended to be construed or to serve as a standard of medical care. Standards of medical care are determined on the basis of all clinical data available for an individual case and are subject to change as scientific knowledge and technology advance and patterns evolve. These parameters of practice should be considered guidelines only. Adherence to them will not ensure a successful outcome in every case, nor should they be construed as including all proper methods of care or excluding other acceptable methods of care aimed at the same results. The ultimate judgment regarding a particular clinical procedure or treatment plan must be made by the psychiatrist in light of the clinical data presented by the patient and the diagnostic and treatment options available.

"Secret" Criteria

The issue of secret criteria has been partially addressed by the Utilization Review Accreditation Council (URAC). URAC has urged the review companies to make their criteria sets available to practitioners and in fact has made this condition one of the criteria for accreditation by URAC. This is an important step forward that clinicians view very positively. The next step is to have criteria sets that the review or managed care company and the practitioners both accept as being clinically sound and helpful as a guide. Criteria sets that are based on guidelines accepted by the profession can meet that goal.

Expertise and Experience of Reviewers

The fifth problem may not be significantly affected by the use of practice guidelines. It is hoped that using the guidelines will result in questions from the reviewer that are more relevant and appropriate. Also, having a common language (based on the guideline) may partially compensate for the reviewer's knowing significantly less about the patient than the practitioner does and perhaps even for the reviewer's not having the same level of expertise or experience as the practitioner does. However, this issue is likely to remain both significant and difficult to resolve.

Use and Misuse of Practice Guidelines

Theoretically, then, practice guidelines may be quite helpful to clinicians in a number of ways. Of course, it is also possible that guidelines can be misused.

Let us take two actual clinical vignettes that demonstrate both how practice guidelines can be misused and also how they can be a help to clinicians in the review process.

Shortly before the practice guideline for eating disorders was approved, the Office of Research at the American Psychiatric Association (where the practice guideline project is housed) received an urgent call. A psychiatrist reported that he had been told by a reviewer that additional inpatient care was not going to be authorized for his patient because the patient should be treated on an outpatient basis. When the psychiatrist asked on what grounds this decision was made, he was told that it was on the basis of the American Psychiatric Association's practice guideline on eating disorders. The guideline had not yet been approved, but apparently the review company had access to a draft of the guideline and was quoting from that draft.

The psychiatrist then obtained a copy of the draft so that he could discuss this matter in more detail with the reviewer. The reviewer had extracted a statement from the guideline that some patients can be treated effectively with psychoanalysis. Extrapolating from that statement, the reviewer told the treating psychiatrist that his patient could be treated on an outpatient basis with psychoanalysis. The reviewer then told the psychiatrist that "this policy does not cover psychoanalysis"!

This clear misuse of a guideline—lifting a sentence out of context or extrapolating from comments in the guideline to unwarranted conclusions—is what clinicians identify as a potential negative effect of the use of guidelines. Fortunately, in this case, when the psychiatrist obtained the guideline, he was able to discuss it with a psychiatrist reviewer; they agreed that this was an erroneous conclusion and a misuse of the guideline, and the review determination was reversed.

Shortly after the guideline on eating disorders was published, a psychiatrist reported that authorization for additional inpatient days had been denied to a patient under his care who had a diagnosis of an eating disorder. The psychiatrist appealed this determination and asked the reviewing psychiatrist to reconsider this case based on principles outlined in the practice guideline. The reviewing psychiatrist agreed to do so and reversed the review determination, and additional inpatient days were authorized.

Conclusion

It is clear that good managed care companies and good clinicians have goals that overlap. Both want the patient to receive treatment that is effective at a cost that is reasonable. Practice guidelines can be the common language that allows informed dialogue about these matters to occur. If these guidelines are to be truly helpful, they must be based on evidence, and they must be accepted by the clinician and the reviewing company. If the guidelines now being developed gain this acceptance, they can become an important part of the evolving health care system and contribute to the effort to increase access to high-quality psychiatric care for individuals with mental illnesses.

Recommended Reading

American Psychiatric Association: Practice guideline for eating disorders. Am J Psychiatry 150 (suppl), February 1993

American Psychiatric Association: Practice guideline for major depressive disorder in adults. Am J Psychiatry 150 (suppl), April 1993

McIntyre JS, Talbott JA: Practice parameters: what they are and why they're needed. Hosp Community Psychiatry 41:1103–1105, 1990

Zarin DA, Pincus HA, McIntyre JS: Practice guidelines. Am J Psychiatry 150:175–177, 1993

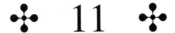
Quality-of-Care Guidelines

The Managed Care View

ALEX R. RODRIGUEZ, M.D.[*]

Clinical standards and guidelines, whether explicit or implicit, are an inherent foundation for the clinical decision-making process. Both form the basis in contemporary health services for clinical training, practice, and monitoring. They have evolved through the course of premodern and modern medicine to reflect both the science and the art of clinical care. In the context of current mental health care in the United States, quality-of-care standards and guidelines now frame clinical decisions that, ideally, should result in the highest quality process and outcome with the lowest possible risk to the patient and in the most cost-effective manner. Developing the broadest public consensus for such standards and guidelines is now one of the major challenges facing professional organizations and payers for health services.

Clinical quality standards and guidelines evolve from a number of sources. Explicit standards and guidelines are those developed by profes-

---

[*]Chief Medical Officer, Preferred Works/Value Health, Wilton, Connecticut; Instructor in Psychiatry, Yale University School of Medicine, New Haven, Connecticut.

sional bodies and publicly promulgated. Implicit guidelines are clinical rule bases that are either commonly accepted by clinicians or individually developed through training and practice and utilized to effect clinical decisions. By definition, a clinical standard is a measure or principle with which aspects of a clinically defined area of practice are compared to estimate the relative quality, quantity, or value of treatment. An example, based on published American Psychiatric Association (APA) standards, would be the expectation that a qualified psychiatrist direct needed physical and psychiatric examinations, assessments, and treatment planning within 24 hours of the admission of a patient to an inpatient unit.

A criterion or guideline would be a test or rule for measuring the relative adherence to a standard. For example, the presence of a physician's note in the medical record within 24 hours of admission, stipulating the details of evaluation and treatment planning, would represent both a mode of adherence to and external monitoring of APA's published professional standard. Cognizance of the standard and criterion allows the clinician to practice in a way that increases the chances of a quality outcome and reduces avoidable risks. Utilization of the criterion and guideline by a professional reviewer would allow focus on the absence or presence of a marker for the standard and attention to any oversights through a process of education.

The APA's evolving definitions of such standards, guidelines, and criteria have been notable in the modern era of medical quality assurance. Its efforts have been instrumental in framing the essential clinical center of "responsible" utilization management activities evolving during the past 25 years. They also represent the hope that science and professionalism will not be rendered irrelevant in light of the dramatic changes that are occurring now in health care funding and delivery systems.

Development of Quality-of-Care Guidelines in Current Mental Health Services

In this chapter, Dr. Gibson notes the evaluation of inappropriate and secret review guidelines in the 1970s by various professional standards review organizations and by the Federal Employee Health Benefit Program. Similarly, numerous other review guidelines and criteria were developed by local ad hoc consultants to a myriad of insurers and third-party administrators across the United States during the 1970s and 1980s. Most of these guidelines were developed from a cost-containment and utilization management perspective. They were oriented toward use by review nurses and physician advisers who were tasked with making decisions about the appropriateness of clinical evaluations and treatments at various levels of care. Many of these review systems lacked both the objective guidelines and the qualified mental health professionals required for the expert determination of "medical (psychological) necessity" called for in the health benefit plan. Medically necessary services are commonly defined as those meeting the following criteria:

✣ They are adequate and essential for the evaluation or treatment of a disease, illness, or condition, as defined by standard diagnostic nomenclatures (*Diagnostic and Statistical Manual of Mental Disorders, 3rd Edition, Revised* or *International Classification of Diseases, 9th Revision, Clinical Modification*).
✣ They can reasonably be expected to improve an individual's condition or level of functioning.
✣ They are in keeping with national standards of professional practice as defined by standard clinical references and valid empirical experience for efficacy of therapies.
✣ They are provided at the most cost-effective level of care.

The institution of a national peer review program for inpatient and outpatient mental health services by the Civilian Health and Medical Program of the Uniformed Services (CHAMPUS) with the assistance of both the APA and the American Psychological Association constituted a watershed event in the evolution of quality-of-care guidelines in the United States. Operating under congressional mandates for accountability regarding quality, risks, and costs, CHAMPUS worked closely with the APA and the American Psychological Association during the late 1970s to develop this first national peer review program. A cornerstone component of this program was the set of clinical criteria upon which peer reviews would be based. Panels of distinguished clinicians developed the first published national consensus criteria for psychiatric and psychological services. The wide dissemination of the criteria substantially affected practitioners' treatment planning nationwide because of both the size and the distribution of the CHAMPUS population and the rapid adaptation of the APA criteria by many Blue Cross–Blue Shield plans and commercial insurance carriers. This popular response to the peer review criteria reflected a de facto affirmation of them as a gold standard for review.

Despite this initial use of the APA criteria, they were not universally embraced by third-party payers, which tended to remain more comfortable with their restrictive in-house criteria. With the rapid growth of private utilization management activities during the 1980s, market pressures caused competing utilization review companies to protect their criteria sets—including those evolved from APA and American Psychological Association manuals—under claims that they represented "proprietary" efforts. Over time, a small number of progressive managed mental health companies either have made their criteria available on inquiry or have published them. Criteria have been made public in response to the growing anger by practitioners about the stacked deck that secret criteria represent in the review process. Mental health professionals rightly believe they should understand the supposedly scientific and professional bases on which their treatment plans are to be evaluated. Notwithstanding the common fears of utilization management organizations that knowledge of review criteria would lead to "gaming" of the review process by providers of care, companies that have made their criteria public have presented no evidence that manipulation of clinical information by providers has been any greater when they possess the review guidelines.

As part of the backlash against secret criteria, practitioners from various medical specialties and mental health disciplines have made organized efforts to require criteria disclosure by means of state or federal law and regulation. More than 20 states now have statutes that require some level of criteria disclosure as part of their licensing regulations. Disclosure of criteria during review (but not publication of these criteria) is required of organizations accredited by the Utilization Review Accreditation Commission, a national body established with the support of various constituencies, including providers (e.g., American Medical Association, American Hospital Association, American Psychiatric Association), payers (e.g., Blue Cross and Blue Shield Association, Health Insurance Association of America, National Association of Manufacturers), consumers (e.g., United Auto Workers), regulators (e.g., National

Association of Insurance Commissioners), and reviewers (e.g., American Managed Care and Review Association) of care.

These efforts have served not only to make the plethora of criteria and guidelines more public, but also to highlight the significant variations among them, particularly with respect to current clinical literature and practices. Such variations have further underscored the need for national consensus criteria that would reflect what is known about the efficacy of psychotherapeutic interventions and levels of care for specific clinical conditions. To their credit, two medical organizations—the APA and the American Society of Addiction Medicine—have published national criteria guidelines for the treatment of psychiatric and substance abuse disorders. These efforts represent the necessary evolution of a unified scientific and clinical basis on which local health services should be provided, reviewed, and reimbursed.

Any national or state health care reforms should embrace the application of such scientifically based and professionally and publicly validated standards and criteria. However, any efforts by professional associations to establish practice or review standards will necessarily have to be open to broader public examination, validation, and modification through a consensus process. The American Society of Addiction Medicine's current efforts to evolve its criteria through field trials and consensus development represent exactly the open and scientific approach that is required. Active participation and acceptance by other professional associations (e.g., the APA), managed care organizations, and payers will be critical for true consensus to occur.

One of the most important developments in the confluence of the quality assurance, utilization review, and consumer movements over the past 20 years is the commitment by medical specialty societies and the federal government to develop practice parameters. In an ambitious initiative supported by the American Medical Association, national medical specialty societies such as the APA and the American Academy of Child and Adolescent Psychiatry are now developing an evolving body of professional consensus for treatment of psychiatric disorders. Increasingly, this process will be buttressed by sensitive, reliable, and valid data on the efficacy of various psychiatric evaluations and treatments, rather than by the predominant "common practice" test characteristic of the traditional professional consensus process.

Practice parameters are a necessary and natural evolution of the quest for clinical definitions of medical necessity. More detailed than screening guidelines and criteria, these parameters fill in gaps for both treating and monitoring clinicians, who must mutually establish how treatment is "adequate and essential" in order for placement of patients in a level of care, specific clinical interventions, and reimbursement to be deemed appropriate. Practice parameters represent to both payers and providers of care an important compendium of clinical observations and opinions gleaned from multiple scientific sources (e.g., texts, monographs, journal articles).

Practitioners have been ambivalent about their support of practice parameters for a number of reasons, primarily because of their fears that payers would use them to arbitrarily restrict reimbursement and that attorneys and litigious patients could invoke them in malpractice proceedings. Thus far, it appears that just the opposite is occurring. Where implemented, practice parameters are both reducing malpractice claims and premiums and leading to fewer appeals generated by differences of opinion about medical necessity.

Because parameters can influence the operational costs of review for payers, many payers are now becoming anxious about the timetable for rollout of parameters by professional associations. Many are pressing for a more ambitious federal initiative, led by agencies such as the Agency for Health Care Policy and Research. Some payers are now starting to develop their own practice parameters. This fact should be of great concern to the APA and the American Academy of Child and Adolescent Psychiatry, which now need to examine development funding and timetables in the context of a rapidly evolving market demand.

Guidelines, Parameters, and Outcomes Management

Given the increasingly close legal ties between treatment and review determinations, a focus on evidence for medical necessity is pressing payers and providers to establish systems that demonstrate the efficacy of medical evaluations and treatments. Thus, the rules of evidence are shifting from reliance on expert opinions, based on subjective conjectures, to the rules of science. As important as research-based diagnostic criteria have been to clinical processes and outcomes, so the evolution of research-based standards, criteria, indicators, thresholds, and parameters is quickly becoming highly relevant to clinical care and review. Health services research is shifting from more traditional academic settings to the front lines of clinical services and managed care. This trend is being fueled by many factors—most notably the social doctrines of equity and risk management—that are important components of health services in a communal society, toward which the United States is definitively evolving.

With limited economic resources, many payers and policymakers are now declaring that rules must be established to equitably allocate and ration health services. In Oregon and other settings, mathematical models are being developed that establish health services' eligibility and payment based on scientific indicators of efficacy. These new organized schemes for outcome management offer much promise. However, they present many potential problems that will need to be addressed, notably the following:

Politicization of Research Models and Data

Despite their good intentions of developing a system for increasing access for uninsured persons, programs such as Oregon Health Decisions have political agendas that influence the real "fairness" of the coverage. The social and economic worth of persons needing high-cost care in a community where they may not live productively (i.e., work and pay taxes) ultimately enters into any scientific equation about efficacy.

Notwithstanding the fact that persons deemed candidates for orthotopic liver transplantation have a survival rate of greater than 70%, Oregon initially calculated that it could not afford such procedures for its Medicaid population. Only after federal pressures were exerted did Oregon embrace the medical necessity of the procedure. The high costs of certain procedures (e.g., bone marrow transplant for breast cancer treatment) and medications (e.g., clozapine) definitely influence payers' policies and review activities. In the coming stages of national health reform, national consensus standards are direly needed to minimize the social and economic agendas that can pervert science, professional ethics, and human compassion.

Integrated Data Systems and the Use of Data

It is now generally accepted that reimbursement of health care expenses in the future will hinge on evidence that specific procedures and treatments are efficacious. Formal technology- and therapeutic-assessment programs have increased in numbers and activities over the past 15 years to meet payers' requirements for scientific evidence that medical and psychological treatments are both clinically effective and cost-effective. Increasingly, managers of such programs have realized that meta-analysis of available scientific data requires large, diverse data bases.

In his call for a national strategic plan for outcome management, Paul Elwood, M.D., has advocated the development of a national data base on clinical and cost outcomes that would integrate the now-disconnected plethora of data files maintained by insurance companies, third-party administrators, and managed care organizations. An undertaking of such magnitude and complexity would require federal leadership in the form of government-provided incentives and financing. Among the areas requiring the most attention would be security systems to protect sensitive individual patient and provider data. The many challenges of developing such a system must be met—and in a "reasonable" time frame (i.e., less than 10 years)—if the nation is ever to have a truly credible base for defining the efficacy of the treatments that will be competing for reimbursements. In turn, future generations of practice parameters, standards, and criteria would emanate from such a consolidated data pool.

The Continuing and Evolving Roles of the Professions

Societies of health care professionals have historically functioned to promote scientific knowledge, education, clinical standards, and ethics. Over time, they have become part of the rich political and business environment in the United States, enticed by the need to represent the economic and other interests of their members. Thus, the APA entered the commercial review business in the 1980s, and the American Psychological Association is now engaged in marketing a managed care plan. Professional associations now routinely make political pronouncements on subjects as diverse as abortion, controversial television shows, and global warming. Some have abandoned the development of practice standards, many are publicly chastised for failing to establish adequate ethical standards and member accountability, and all seem to bicker endlessly with one another about the turf of patient care.

Associations of mental health professionals must both increase their commitments to their traditional roles (particularly development of standards) and learn to work together for the common defense of the endangered mental health benefit. Current efforts by the National Mental Health Leadership Forum to influence the adequacy and parity of mental health benefits within the context of national health care reform are a good start. As much as—or more than—any other single commitment, collaboration to promote and develop national mental health practice and review standards will better serve both the economic interests of association members and the health status of patients.

The Brave New World of Standardized Practice

The changes in health care that are now confronting practitioners are truly profound. As such, they are both frightening and exciting—frightening because they are wrenching independent judgment and control away from the clinician and exciting because they offer such hope for care that is better integrated, coordinated, meaningful to patients, and cost-effective. Although some managed care organizations are abusive to providers, arbitrarily restrict patients' access to necessary care, and establish administrative barriers to benefit authorization and payment, others are garnering high marks from providers and patients for their clinical sensitivity and objectivity, administrative efficiencies, and contributions to effective care. Such programs promote dialogue, trust, and professionalism in their relationships with providers and their associations. They realize that their success in attracting and retaining benefit plans as customers depends on high patient and provider satisfaction, as well as the ability to structure local treatment systems so that they reliably deliver high-quality, cost-effective care. Establishing a consensus about the standards of care and review used to make treatment and benefit authorization decisions will be a major step toward achieving that goal.

Professional associations such as the APA will need to affirm this goal as one that serves their members and to increase their efforts in developing national consensus standards and criteria. Practitioners' fears about a standards-driven system of "cookbook medicine" will need to be assuaged by professional leadership that affirms a scientific approach to treatment and that educates its members about the benefits of a standardized practice. Although payers and patients are willing to allow providers some time to change their current habits of clinical decision making, they are impatient for treatment that is better explained, coordinated, and integrated. In the brave new world of managed care, time will be marked more rapidly by those who see an urgent need for change.

The Clinician's View

ROBERT W. GIBSON, M.D.[*]

Attempts to improve the quality of care before 1965 focused on education standards for physicians, procedures for determining the outcome of practice, and standards for measuring a hospital environment. Little or no attention was directed toward the specific practice patterns of physicians and other professionals. Few systematic attempts were made to create quality-of-care guidelines.

By deliberate design, the enactment of Medicare dramatically increased the access to health care for persons over 65 years of age, medically indigent persons, and several groups with special needs. The annual cost of health care in 1965 was only about $40 billion, claiming just 5.9% of the gross national product (GNP). Making health care accessible to tens of millions of people fueled an increase in costs that far exceeded all predictions.

The cost-containment provisions of Medicare included requirements

[*]President Emeritus, The Sheppard and Enoch Pratt Hospital, Baltimore, Maryland.

for utilization review to determine the appropriateness and medical necessity of care. Under Medicare, utilization review relied on implicit standards applied by the providers themselves. Understandably, such utilization review had little impact on cost or on patterns of practice. Indeed, the opening sentence of Title XVIII of the Social Security Amendments of 1965, otherwise known as Medicare, provided this reassurance: "Nothing in this title shall be construed to authorize any federal officer or employee to exercise any supervision or control over the practice of medicine or the manner in which medical services are provided . . . ." So much for political promises.

Dissatisfied by the failure of utilization review to limit spending, Congress passed The Social Security Amendments of 1972, which established professional standards review organizations. This action led to a collaborative effort by 30 national specialty societies to generate criteria sets (guidelines) that encompassed the majority of diagnostic criteria and established definitions according to diagnosis for indications for admission, diagnostic procedures, treatment modalities, and review periods.

Within this same time frame (late 1960s and early 1970s), private insurers expanded their benefits to cover services for mental illness. As overall costs of health care rose and competition increased, private insurers tried to control costs. A notable example occurred in 1972 when the Federal Employees Blue Cross Plan projected a single-year loss of some $60 million.

As retroactive denials for psychiatric treatment occurred at an alarming rate, it was discovered that Federal Employees Blue Cross reviewers were using guidelines that favored the use of psychosurgery, insulin therapy, electroconvulsive treatment, and high-dosage drug therapy. Treatments such as psychotherapy (both individual and group), rehabilitative services, and lower-dose drug therapy were dismissed as adjunctive. Claims reviewers denied thousands of claims on the basis that they did not meet these blatantly inappropriate standards for quality and medical necessity. It became clear that guidelines established by payers were not open to public scrutiny and were designed for cost control, not to improve psychiatric care or the mental health delivery system.

In response to the ominous threats to psychiatric practice, the American Psychiatric Association's (APA's) leaders initiated a collaborative effort to develop operational guidelines that reflected current psychiatric practice. These guidelines were combined with procedures described in the APA's *Manual of Psychiatric Peer Review* and became the keystone of a nationwide system.

I considered this initiative so critical that I made it the central theme of my 1977 APA Presidential Address, urging that psychiatrists be made a part of the review system so that: 1) clinical judgments would reflect current psychiatric concepts; 2) meaningful studies could be conducted by psychiatrists with specialized clinical competence; 3) standards and criteria would be established, refined, and modified by the profession; 4) standards and criteria would be open to public scrutiny; 5) and findings could be used to improve psychiatric care as well as to control abuse and unnecessary expenditures. It is my belief that claims review should become a part of our professional quality assurance system—a resource contributing to the improvement of mental health care.

Under a contract with the Civilian Health and Medical Program of the Uniformed Services (CHAMPUS), the APA expanded its efforts by developing an extensive peer review system to determine the medical necessity and appropriateness of services provided to CHAMPUS beneficiaries. Under this system, APA reviewers addressed not only the reasonableness of expenditures, but also the quality and appropriateness of the treatment rendered. Their findings were presented in a collegial and consultative tone rather than a punitive and regulatory one. On balance, this APA system fulfilled the five criteria outlined in my 1977 address. It was still perceived, however, by many payers and providers as a tool for cost control rather than for quality assurance.

In time, several concerns surfaced. Despite reductions in length of hospital stays and outpatient visits, payers wanted still further cost reductions. Treating professionals were angered by denials of their claims even though these denials had been made by highly qualified peers. A new breed of managed care organizations went directly to large employers and promised dramatic cost reductions through carve outs and management of the psychiatric benefits provided to their employees. Faced with escalating health care costs, this was an offer few employers could refuse. This constellation of events highlighted the conflicting and overlapping interests of government, providers, professionals, insurers, and consumers.

The Goals of Health Care

These conflicting and overlapping interests can be subsumed under three major goals: improved access to care, improved quality of care, and control of costs. In the almost three decades since the enactment of Medicare, we have never achieved all three goals. Indeed, it can be argued that we have failed to achieve any of these goals. With 37 million people uninsured, we do not have universal access. Quality often falls short of our professional aspirations. The costs of health care, as measured by the percentage of consumption of the GNP, have increased from 6% to 14% since the enactment of Medicare.

Access, quality, and cost are the end products of a complex interplay of the interests of consumers, providers, and payers. The overriding concern of consumers has been access. Providers have focused on their own definitions of quality for the individual patient, with little regard for the overall mental health delivery system. Payers have become preoccupied by costs as the escalation of health care has reached crisis proportions; managed care activities sometimes have compromised access and dismissed quality as unmeasurable.

Health Care Reform: Why Now?

As early as 1970, government leaders asserted that there would be a breakdown in the delivery of health care unless immediate, concentrated action was taken. There was even talk of some form of national health insurance. But the steps taken to solve the crisis created by the competing demands of access, quality, and cost were at best palliative and at worst driven by self-interest. Why? In my judgment, government and professional leaders failed to undertake major health care reform over the past two decades because there was no political crisis corresponding to the perceived health care crisis.

During the 1992 presidential campaign, health care emerged as a major political issue. The magnitude of the health care expenditures had finally caught the attention of government leaders, just as business leaders in the 1980s turned to managed care when they realized that employee health care costs were affecting the bottom line of their companies. Now, government leaders have concluded that the deficit problem cannot be solved without dealing with runaway health care costs.

Any attempt to achieve universal access to adequate health care by covering the estimated 37 million uninsured persons in the United States will ignite an escalation in health care costs comparable to that seen when Medicare was enacted. With 30 years of failure to control costs, it is clear that radical changes will be required if health care reform is to fulfill the competing goals of access, quality, and cost control. If one of these three goals is achieved by compromising either of the other two, we will have health care destruction, not health care reform.

In the best of all worlds, one might hope that the conflicting and overlapping interests of the consumer, the provider, and the payer would effect a balance among the competing goals of access, quality, and cost control. Unfortunately, experience has demonstrated that this balance is seldom achieved and that any flaws and inequities will be magnified in mental health care.

Access

The consumer might be expected to take the lead in demanding universal access. But the stigma and denial associated with mental illness have been serious barriers. Persons who have suffered a mental illness are often reluctant to expose themselves by coming forward.

Those individuals thus far spared do not expect that they will ever need psychiatric treatment. More recently, advocacy groups have pressed for better services; understandably, however, they have often concentrated their efforts on their particular personal concern.

Providers have articulated the need for increased access based on their clinical experience and research studies. But the views of providers have been discounted as self-serving and have been fragmented by professional turf battles. Such disputes make it easy for decision makers to do nothing while waiting for the experts to get their act together.

The major payers—federal and state governments, not-for-profit and commercial insurers, and employers—have all taken the initiative to expand access. They have made services available to underserved populations and have increased the scope of services provided. When costs have escalated, however,the payers have been forced to balance mental health care costs against other expenditures. In the absence of a strong demand, benefits have been cut.

Quality

Providers have failed to define quality in objective and measurable terms. Opposing schools of thought (e.g., biological versus dynamic and inpatient versus outpatient) have made consensus difficult. Early efforts to develop guidelines were attacked by many practitioners as an intrusion on the autonomy of the individual. Too often, these guidelines were expected to protect professional practice rather than to set true measures of care that could be targets of excellence.

The typical consumer has a difficult time in judging quality as defined by professionals, because consumers look for satisfaction rather than quality. Clearly, there is a significant overlap between these two characteristics of care, but they are by no means the same. A growing number of consumers who are well informed (sometimes because of personal experience) have become a potent force to improve quality.

The big payers for mental health services—the government, the insurers, and more recently the employers—first accepted the judgments of providers. However, as costs have increased, they have begun to ask not only whether mental health treatment is necessary, but also whether it is efficient and efficacious and whether the outcomes warrant the investment. These have become their proxy measures for quality in contrast to professional standards of clinical practice.

Cost

Without question, the payers have been the movers and shakers in the cost-control arena. In my opinion, however, most of the early attempts at cost controls were a somewhat academic exercise to fulfill a legislative requirement or management expectation. As long as the bills could be comfortably paid through taxes, insurance premiums, or corporate revenues, there was no compelling need to become serious about cost control. But the situation has been changed by federal and state deficits, fierce competition among insurers, and falling corporate revenues. All health care expenditures have been targeted, and mental health care in particular has been a casualty. Why mental health care? Again, the reasons are lack of objective measures of quality, lack of understanding of mental illness, and—even now—the effect of stigma.

Consumers have been insulated from cost control of general medical and surgical services by government- and employer-sponsored benefit plans. The users of mental health services have been somewhat more cost conscious because of higher up-front deductibles, higher coinsurance, and annual and lifetime benefit limits. These cost constraints have influenced the decisions of individual users, yet they have produced little significant systemic change in the mental health care delivery system.

Providers of mental health services in the 1970s and early 1980s made some modest efforts to contain costs. Since the mid-1980s, the pressures of managed care review have forced shorter inpatient stays and reduction of the number of outpatient visits. Providers have become important players in cost control by restructuring services, by more efficiently using staff resources, and by developing out-of-hospital alternatives. Regrettably, the constraints imposed by managed care have led to the denial and withholding of needed services.

Health Care Reform

On balance, I fear that the conflicting concerns of consumers, providers, and payers prevent them from being effective marketplace forces that will provide an even-handed or optimal solution to achieving the goal of universal access to mental health care services of adequate quality at an affordable cost. At the federal level, administration and congressional leaders who orchestrate health care reform must deal at the macro level with access, quality, and cost control.

The administration has articulated clearly that the goals of health care reform include universal access to care while containing, or even reducing, overall costs. Providing coverage for the 37 million uninsured persons at an estimated cost of $30–$90 billion annually without increasing costs will inevitably impose serious pressure on quality.

The lack of a uniformly accepted definition makes quality particularly vulnerable. The Department of Health, Education and Welfare, in the *Forward Plan for Health FY 1977–1981*, described quality care as treatment that 1) meets professionally recognized standards; 2) is clinically efficacious, safe, and cost-effective; and 3) satisfies the patient. Managed care providers have already taken the lead in deciding what they consider to be cost-effective treatment—sometimes with and sometimes without any explicitly stated standards and criteria. The APA has made a major commitment to the development of practice guidelines that go far beyond the earlier standards, which focused on admissions and continued-stay criteria. These new practice guidelines were created in response to new concerns about the quality of data and the process used to determine "appropriate" or "reimbursable" care. The goal is " . . . that the psychiatric profession should take the lead in describing the best treatments and the range of appropriate treatments available to patients with mental illness" (American Psychiatric Association 1993, p. 2).

I believe that the most effective way to preserve quality against the pressures of increased access and cost reduction is to blend the emerging APA guidelines with the cost-containment efforts of the managed care communities. The APA's guidelines will provide the benchmark for clinical practice needed to determine 1) the resources required for the type and frequency of services rendered, 2) the necessary qualifications of the professionals, 3) the duration of treatment, and 4) the settings in which services must be provided. Such a two-part definition would provide an interface between quality and cost.

In my judgment, guidelines that combine quality and cost can be created most effectively and credibly by the professional and managed care communities working in concert. Guidelines created by the APA and managed care professionals would allay the fears that when providers ask for quality, they want a blank check, and when payers ask for cost control, they want the dollars to dictate the type and quality of treatment. Most importantly, this process would follow Peter Drucker's advice that the best way to predict the future is to create it.

Reference

American Psychiatric Association: Practice guidelines. Am J Psychiatry 150:2, February 1993

❖ 12 ❖

Ethical Issues Under Managed Care

The Managed Care View

JAMES E. SABIN, M.D.[*]

This condensed version of a representative dialogue from the clinical front lines illustrates many of the central ethical issues in managed care practice. How many readers of this book have not heard or participated in an exchange like the following?

Clinician: This patient is psychotic and disorganized. I think he needs immediate inpatient hospitalization.

Care manager: I think he could be handled in day treatment with rapid medication and a highly structured program.

Thus far, neither party has proposed anything unreasonable. Both clinical recommendations are potentially consistent with good practice.

---

[*]Associate Director, Teaching Programs, Harvard Community Health Plan; Assistant Clinical Professor of Psychiatry, Harvard Medical School, Boston, Massachusetts.

The ethically crucial issue is what happens next. We would hope to see a process of cooperative negotiation and clinical planning. However, like our patients, we mental health professionals often deal with conflict by distortion, splitting, and passionate moralizing. It would not be surprising, therefore, if the vignette continued as follows:

Clinician: The family is coming apart at the seams and can't handle him at home. Everyone is so anxious his symptoms will only get worse. In the past he got suicidal when his family was scared and that will happen again if we force day hospitalization on them.

Care manager: Isn't it really just the opposite? Sticking him into 24-hour care will undermine his ability to cope with his illness and reinforce the family's belief that they have to extrude him as soon as the psychosis appears.

Clinician: I can't go along with the idea of day treatment—it isn't safe. [Clinician's thought: All this care manager worries about is saving money for the insurer—he doesn't give a ***bleep*** about quality.]

Care manager: I can't authorize inpatient treatment—it isn't indicated and it will be regressive. [Care manager's thought: All this clinician worries about is making things easier for himself and filling beds in the hospital—he doesn't give a ***bleep*** about quality.]

This all-too-frequent form of failed collaboration exemplifies four common ethical issues in managed care practice:

First, if the clinician is truly claiming to *know* that without 24-hour hospital care the patient will become suicidal, he is displaying a narcissistic denial of the inherent uncertainty of clinical prediction. Scientific humility acknowledges uncertainty and works with it. Professional narcissism simply denies it. If the clinician does not mean to be claiming omniscience, however, he is—perhaps unwittingly—speaking with duplicity and must be suspected of using pseudocertainty to "game" the system to obtain approval for hospitalization.

Second, instead of seeing the exchange as a clinical disagreement to be explored in a reasoned manner, the clinician interprets the care manager's perspective as an irreconcilable difference in fundamental values. His commitment to his own preferred treatment approach is more theological than clinical. The clinician assumes that the care manager is unconcerned about quality because he does not endorse inpatient hospitalization. Like a religious fundamentalist, he holds that anyone who questions his belief about what needs to be done is showing a deeply unethical attitude.

Third, if the care manager invoked the regressive potential of inpatient care as a *possibility,* he would be on strong clinical ground. Hospitalization can undermine adaptive efforts and reinforce the family's dysfunctional beliefs about the patient. However, when he says it will *certainly* be regressive, he too is lapsing into narcissistic denial of uncertainty or his own version of "gaming"—just as the clinician did. Much as clinicians may exaggerate symptoms to obtain approval for more-restrictive (and costly) modes of treatment, care managers may exaggerate the regressive potential of these same modes to rationalize denying approval.

Finally, the care manager has not sought to develop an alliance with the clinician. He makes no effort to ascertain whether the clinician has the skills needed to carry out a more efficient intervention. His recommendation is too vague to be useful. Which day program? How can the clinician address his concerns about the family? What should be done first? Day treatment will remain a dubious approach until these questions are addressed.

I could easily expand on the ethical problems in this failure of managed care, but it is more useful to return to the dialogue to suggest what successful collaboration would look like. Then, rather than fighting ethical fires and excoriating each other, the clinician and the care manager can act in the spirit of quality improvement and ask which interventions may promote ethically admirable managed care.

Clinician: I see your point and I am sure you see mine. Suppose we plan for a short inpatient admission. I can probably get him into day treatment in a week.

Care manager: That's a reasonable idea, but I think we have a good chance of getting the same results for less cost. I know day treatment puts more strain on you and the family, but we can probably find ways of making it tolerable. Suppose we use a holding bed tonight so you can help the patient and the family calm down, start day treatment tomorrow, have the home care nurse make a visit, and see how it goes?

Clinician: I prefer my idea, but I think I can live with yours. [Clinician's thought: "I'm anxious about this approach but the care manager is fair, and if it doesn't work we can always bring the patient in."]

Care manager: I'll check in 3 days to see how it is going. You know how to contact me if there is a problem. [Care manager's thought: I don't think we really need the overnight bed, but the clinician is trying and learning so I think the plan is OK."]

This version of the dialogue is more than a Pollyannaish fantasy. This kind of collaboration already occurs. However, in order to make it the norm of practice rather than the exception, clinicians, managed care professionals, and society itself will have to make some difficult changes in their fundamental outlook.

When clinicians take what I call a "theological" attitude towards their preferred schools of treatment, they do so for strong reasons. Methodologies work better when the clinician conveys firm conviction about the potency of the approach. Quite apart from the specific cognitive-behavioral, psychodynamic, systemic, or pharmacological impacts of a technique, belief in the approach and faithful adherence to its teachings improve outcomes, presumably by adding "nonspecific" or placebo factors to the active ingredients of the treatment itself.

Further, and equally important, belief also reduces anxiety for the physician. In *The Silent World of Doctor and Patient,* Jay Katz documented just how reluctant we clinicians are to acknowledge uncertainty to ourselves and discuss it with patients. When confronted with human suffering and need, we are much more comfortable to "know for sure" what to do than to have hypotheses and educated guesses. Historically, the healer was a religious figure. Hippocrates was a cult leader, not simply a physician. Religions are based on certainties, not hypotheses.

As a foundation for ethical practice, clinicians need to learn how to evince the traditional healing attitude of hope and positive expectations for the treatment while eschewing a fundamentalist or theological attachment to their approaches to care. In business, successful managers are not theological about their methods. They focus on producing outcomes, not on techniques, dogmas, or professional prerogatives. Clinicians need to develop some of the skills and values of excellent managers.

In the past, it was common to hear clinicians discuss whether the patient was a "candidate" for a particular treatment. Thinking about care this way reflects a failure of professional ethics. Clinical education must provide students with flexible attitudes and a broader base of skills so they can adapt their techniques to the demands of efficiency and meet the needs of a wider range of patients. Treatments are candidates for patients, not vice versa.

Clinical training traditionally centers on the care of the individual patient. In a country that sacrifices so many other basic social goods to pay for health care, this focus is too narrow. In addition to emphasizing *fiduciary* commitment to the welfare of the individual patient, clinical training and professional associations need to foster a comparable commitment to *stewardship* of society's resources. When the care manager said "I think we have a good chance of getting the same results for less cost," he was evincing the combination of fiduciary and stewardship concerns that fosters ethically admirable managed care.

The care manager's basic clinical intuition is correct. We do have the expertise to maintain standards of quality and reduce costs, but doing so will require a fundamental change in the public's attitude toward limits. It is not reasonable to expect clinicians—whether moved by their own allegiance to stewardship values or prodded by third-party reviewers and capitation arrangements—to take the lead in educating the public about hard choices if politicians continue to run for cover when health care allocation and the possibility of rationing surface. Clinicians and managed care advocates need to join together to force political and professional leaders to create public understanding of what limits mean in health care. Society simply cannot have a fully free choice of clinicians, methods of treatment, and hospitals; a high-technology style of practice; and no queuing—while containing costs at the same time.

The reader may wonder what these somewhat abstract considerations of fiduciary and stewardship values imply for frontline clinical practice.

The answer has more to do with heart than mind. Clinicians will put their hearts into improved efficiency and cost containment only if they see that their efforts expand access and benefits or promote other social goods. The following (disguised) example shows that when clinicians are able to integrate fiduciary and stewardship concerns, they are able to foster an ethically sound therapeutic alliance with their patients.

> Dr. Jones was treating Mr. G., a patient with relatively mild atypical depression and chronic Axis II pathology. An antidepressant regimen was well established and required little attention. Mr. G. used appointments to review his chronically turbulent personal life and to seek insight, advice, and guidance. He valued the appointments a great deal, and Dr. Jones believed that Mr. G. did indeed derive benefit from these appointments. In the health maintenance organization (HMO) setting, Dr. Jones could not see Mr. G. more than once a month for 45 minutes. Mr. G. protested, "I will improve faster if I see you more often." Dr. Jones wasn't sure whether or not this was so. He said, "You may well be right. If we had 10 national experts here, I'm sure many would agree with you, though probably not all. But the HMO budgets psychiatrists' time to make the insurance premium go as far as possible. That means I can only see you once a month. Let's see how we can use the time most productively."

For costs to be managed in an ethical manner, reviewers, clinicians, and patients will have to learn to talk candidly about resource limits the way Dr. Jones and Mr. G. did in this case example. Unfortunately, such conversations do not happen often at present. Trade-offs between cost and quality are not unethical in themselves, but keeping the process secret is. In this situation, Dr. Jones was not sure whether limiting Mr. G.'s psychiatric visits to 45 minutes a month represented "trimming fat" or withholding potentially beneficial treatment (rationing). There are no outcome data specific enough to provide a dose-response curve for Mr. G.'s treatment. Dr. Jones acknowledged uncertainty by invoking the hypothetical panel of experts. He did not fall into a theological stance of pseudocertainty, whether by assailing the HMO for a "takeover of mental health practice by business interests, with devastating effects on patients, practitioners, and the professions" ("The Trauma of Managed Mental Health Care" 1993, p. A14) or by asserting that more intensive treatment would harm Mr. G. by "creating dependency."

In the case of Mr. G., the contentious issue involves withholding a resource (more frequent visits) that the patient wants. The ethical situation is more difficult when economic considerations push for use of a treatment that the patient opposes, as in the following case example:

> Mr. H. suffered from bipolar disorder, partly controlled by lithium carbonate. Over 2 weeks his sleep became erratic. There were possible early psychotic features in his thought. In the past, manic episodes had required hospitalization and neuroleptic medication. Dr. Jones reviewed the situation with Mr. H., emphasizing that if they used neuroleptic medication now they might be doing it unnecessarily and would be adding slightly to the risk of tardive dyskinesia and other side effects. A delay in starting medication might result in an otherwise avoidable hospitalization. Mr. H. unequivocally wanted to minimize the risk of hospitalization, so they agreed to add the neuroleptic agent.
>
> Ms. I.'s clinical condition was very much the same as that of Mr. H., except that Ms. I. was extremely negative about using neuroleptics and neither she nor her family was at all dismayed at the prospect of hospitalization.

What stance should we ask Dr. Jones to take with Ms. I.? Insofar as not using neuroleptic medication increases the likelihood of an otherwise avoidable hospitalization, Dr. Jones and Ms. I. would be taking risks with other people's money. Should Dr. Jones follow fiduciary values and act as the patient's advocate, or should he be guided by stewardship concerns and speak for the HMO subscribers whose premiums are at increased risk without neuroleptic use? I believe the ethically correct answer is "both."

Clinicians, administrators, and the public need to struggle with questions like these before they arise as frontline ethical crises. Here is how I would have Dr. Jones respond:

> Dr. Jones explained that the HMO tries to limit hospital use to what is absolutely necessary, but acknowledged the importance of Ms. I.'s preferences. They agreed to add clonazepam to help with sleep and arranged for daily telephone contact to monitor her status. They planned to review the question of neuroleptics again if her clinical status deteriorated further.

Ethically admirable managed care requires a constructive level of tension between clinicians (who are closest to the patient and therefore best able to identify and advocate for fiduciary concerns) and administrators or reviewers (who can speak best for stewardship considerations). Both voices are needed. During the past 10–20 years, unmanaged fee-for-service reimbursement encouraged clinicians and hospitals to neglect stewardship, as evidenced by unsustainable cost inflation. Managed care has emerged as the centerpiece of our national effort to correct this ethical imbalance. Clinicians will only regain professional autonomy when they accept responsibility for stewardship of society's resources.

In the Preamble to the *Principles of Medical Ethics* of the American Medical Association and the American Psychiatric Association, we find the following statement: "As a member of this profession, a physician must recognize responsibility not only to patients *but also to society . . .* " (emphasis added). Unfortunately, neither the annotations to the *Principles of Medical Ethics* nor the *Opinions of the Ethics Committee on the Principles of Medical Ethics* clarify the nature of the psychiatrist's responsibility to society. Professional leadership has not yet gone beyond lip service to the stewardship component of professional ethics. As a result, many clinicians see only that managed care does indeed create new ethical problems, while altogether failing to recognize its importance in helping our nation solve the very serious old ethical problem of inadequate stewardship.

The central ethical question in future managed care practice will be how to decide when proposed interventions warrant their cost. In order to collaborate in developing creative solutions to this fundamental question, clinicians, managed care professionals, and the public will need a shared ethical framework. Once we finally recognize and truly accept the need to integrate fiduciary and stewardship values and to work constructively with the inevitable tensions that arise, we will be able to get down to practical implementation of ethical approaches—the way the clinician and care manager did in their second try at resolving the issue of inpatient care versus day treatment.

Reference

Edward J, Shore K: The trauma of managed mental health care (letter). The New York Times, February 15, 1993, p A14

The Clinician's View

STEVEN S. SHARFSTEIN, M.D., M.P.A.[*]

As a physician and provider of mental health services, my main ethical obligation is to the patient. The patient comes first, and this requires not only "doing no harm," but also making secondary my own economic and other needs and priorities, as the Hippocratic Oath states. The issues, of course, are complex, and often there are a variety of conflicting questions—especially when the patient's view of his or her needs and my own views, which reflect treatment standards and community practice, conflict. This conflict becomes especially problematic when the cost issues are brought directly into the doctor-patient relationship, and trade-offs in quality and access are expected in the transaction between doctor and patient. If my ethical obligation is to the patient, cost issues must also be secondary. Here is the conflict with managed care.

Managed care is fundamentally an effort to contain costs within some boundaries of quality and access. At the present time, managed care is imposed from the outside, but that situation is changing as payers contract directly with preferred providers and health maintenance organizations (HMOs) that are able to demonstrate the ability to contain costs within a clinical consensus on access and quality. Currently, most of the focus is on telephone review or utilization management. Soon it will be on whether I can resolve my ethical conflicts in the context of a very specific contract with a public or private managed care vendor.

Issues for Today

At the present time, when a managed care reviewer is on the 800 line, I struggle with that reviewer to achieve a consensus on medical necessity

[*]Medical Director and Chief Executive Officer, The Sheppard and Enoch Pratt Hospital, Baltimore, Maryland; Clinical Professor of Psychiatry, University of Maryland Medical School, Baltimore, Maryland.

and appropriateness. That requires the reviewer to share the criteria and guidelines he or she uses in allowing my patient access to care. Surely the openness of dialogue can only occur when these parameters, standards, and guidelines are fully open and not secret. If there are computer logarithms and specific written expectations in terms of need to hospitalize, number of days, and number of visits, these all must be shared. It's when I'm notified that the criteria are "secret" that immediately I detect the aroma of ethical trouble.

The cordiality and tact of the dialogue between myself and the managed care reviewer are critical aspects. Mutual respect, even in the face of a clinical disagreement, allows dialogue to take place. If over time that respect can grow, it is possible to diverge from criteria when an individual patient requires it and there is a good clinical rationale to do so. I have experienced this positive aspect of utilization management, but unfortunately it's been rare.

The outside review of care should have all the components of a good clinical consultation; however, from an ethical perspective, it should be more than that. Utilization management of patient care requires a certain amount of risk sharing, especially when patients may be a danger to themselves or others. In the context of managing care, it is important that there is an openly acknowledged sharing of responsibility for these clinical risks. I wonder about the ethics of denying care and then washing one's hands of any responsibility for untoward consequences when the patient is discharged because of economics and signs out against medical advice, and a fragile treatment plan is disrupted. Some managed care companies do, in fact, assume some risk. They will directly interview the patient with the clinical team present and thereby share clinical risk. In the context of these difficult clinical decisions, there is a legitimate gray zone in deciding on the degree of suicidality in a particular patient.

A further issue in the context of moving patients more rapidly out of the hospital is whether my patients can access the continuum of care through utilization management or the managed care system. Unfortunately, much of the denial of hospitalization has been a form of deinstitutionalization of the insured or middle class. The availability and accessibility of alternative services such as day treatment, more intensive outpatient services, and home care have been limited. The exception is when the managed care company is entitled to flex the benefits and provide for high-cost case management. In those instances, there is a congruence of patient need, economics, and the managed care process that for me feels ethically correct.

Another important issue is whether the managed care system allows continuity of treatment with an individual provider if that provider is not part of a new contract for care. Too often, treatment is totally disrupted when a new group of providers is introduced in the middle of treatments for patients who already have a therapeutic alliance with their own practitioner. There are then intense issues related to abandonment that take on an ethical aspect.

On my end of the ethical continuum, it's critical that I am clear, open, and honest about the clinical signs and symptoms, the impairment I am trying to ameliorate, the rationale of my treatment strategies, and my clinical objectives. I hope that my honesty is rewarded with respect for and consideration of the fact that I am ultimately responsible for the care of my patient. Even if the managed care company is willing to share some of the responsibility for the decision about continuing or denying benefits, it is important that my discussions with utilization managers have a baseline of honesty.

Unfortunately, in some instances, the reviewer on the other end of the phone assumes dishonesty on my part. He or she assumes that I am a lying, conniving provider attempting to line my pockets with the scarce resources of a company's insurance plan. This innuendo creeps into the dialogue and contaminates our important discussion. If one participant in the telephone conversation assumes mendacity, an ethically correct managed care decision cannot be made.

Finally, it is important that I have the time to treat my patients. The concern I have with the time-consuming review, the forms to fill out, the telephone calls to be returned, and the records to copy is that I am becoming an advocate or salesman, a clerk, and an accountant. I did not go to medical school or to a residency training in psychiatry to become a bureaucrat. This may be an efficiency issue, multiplied many thousands of times in terms of the administrative waste in American medicine, but for me it is also an ethical issue because this time is taken away from my patients.

Issues for Tomorrow

In the current era, care of patients is moving toward prepaid group practice and capitation and away from fee-for-service medicine. Many more Americans are enrolling in HMOs or receive their care through preferred providers. As a provider, I must decide which organizations to join and which to avoid. These decisions present a whole new set of ethical dilemmas and considerations.

The conflicts of interest generated by managed care require new obligations on my part with regard to my patients. For example, I should fully disclose to my patients any financial arrangements that may tend to limit the care offered to them or contractual provisions which I agree to that may restrict referral or treatment. If patients choose to participate in such a plan, they should be aware of these restrictions at the time of their enrollment. The managed care plan should disclose to patients enrolled in the plan any contractual agreements that may tend to limit diagnostic and therapeutic alternatives. Nonetheless, I should inform my patient of medically appropriate treatment options whether or not this coverage is part of their contractual agreement or is within the cost expectations of the HMO or preferred provider organization (PPO). The financial incentives involved in my enrollment in an HMO or PPO should not influence my judgment about the necessary and appropriate therapeutic alternatives.

When there are risk-sharing arrangements designed to deter excess utilization, any incentive payments to me should be based on the performance of a group of my colleagues rather than on my individual performance, and there should be a sufficient delay before these incentives come into play. For example, at least a year should pass before such bonus incentives are paid—to deal with rehospitalization rates and other outcomes that show the untoward impact of reduced utilization. Surely, we should encourage the use of the least expensive care setting as long as services can be provided safely and effectively with no determent to quality.

Preferred provider systems or carve outs can sometimes impair the continuity of a patient's care across different treatment settings. The use of high-cost case management has come into play in these situations, and it is important that the primary provider has a critical role in the development of alternative treatment plans for a patient with complicated chronic illness.

Another area of potential ethical concern is patient stealing. As managed care moves from a utilization management approach to a preferred provider approach, patients may be transferred from a nonnetwork clinician to an in-network clinician. The previously discussed continuity-of-care question is only one potential ethical concern. The other occurs when an in-network clinician is asked to consult on a particular case and ends up referring that case into his or her practice. This type of shift can create ethical problems for the in-network provider, who may be accused of stealing the patient.

All of the above ethical concerns can involve questions of fiduciary relationship and responsibility, "double-agentry" issues that have been a long-standing problem for psychiatry in the military and state systems. The conflicts occur when we move from fee-for-service medicine, where the incentive is to do more, to managed care, where the incentive is to do less.

Confidentiality is key and should be protected. In our managed care era, one can become completely cynical about confidentiality. So much information is being passed across 800 telephone lines; entire records are being photocopied and sent off; and clinicians from managed care companies come directly to hospitals and outpatient facilities to examine records, see staff, and even interview the patients. As a result, it's hard to maintain or sustain a critical ethical dimension of practice—the sanctity of a confidential doctor-patient relationship. Yet despite the accountability issues, it is important that confidentiality be protected to the extent possible. Breaches of confidentiality should be thoroughly pursued via the applicable state laws as well as the ethics processes of the various professional associations. Shame, stigma, and distrust are still associated with psychiatric care. These get magnified many times when confidentiality is breached and patients and families become humiliated by the improper divulgence of extremely sensitive information.

Economic incentives should not take the form of kickbacks, bounties, fraud, commissions from savings, and so forth. There is disproportionate power in the delivery of medical and psychiatric care. The providers know much more than the consumers do. Treatment is too expensive for most patients and families to pay out of pocket. They need third-party payments. Our ethics define us as a profession and legitimize our ability to deliver needed treatment. The managed care system must recognize and respect the importance of these ethics. The principle of the patient coming first should be the beacon of light by which these issues are re-solved.

Section V

A Family Perspective

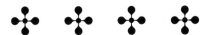

Managed Care and Mental Illness

LAURIE M. FLYNN[*]

"I know what managed care means to mental illness," says Ms. J. "To my family it has meant financial devastation and near ruin. Several of us have long-term mental illnesses, and although my husband works for the federal government and we pay dearly for high-option coverage, we have not been protected from a close brush with losing our home. The reason is simple—most managed care companies simply try to reduce access to treatment. They push you out of services long before you can stand on your own two feet, so middle-class families like mine spend down all their savings, use up any discretionary income they may have in order to cover what managed care refuses to provide."

"Would managed care companies try to discharge cancer patients from the hospital before they have completed their chemotherapy? Do they deny lifesaving medications to people with heart disease? I wonder why mental illness is so often targeted for cost containment."

---

[*]Executive Director of the National Alliance for the Mentally Ill (NAMI), based in Arlington, Virginia. NAMI is a national grassroots family and consumer organization advocating on behalf of persons with severe psychiatric disorders.

As Ms. J.'s personal story clearly indicates, National Alliance for the Mentally Ill (NAMI) families and consumers have had experiences with managed care and mental illness that can be described as difficult at best. We do not challenge the need for controlling costs and managing patient care effectively—it is just that we may have a different definition of how that management should be focused. NAMI families believe that the result of managed care should be provision of what is needed to achieve the best health outcome for the patient. What we see in reality, at least with mental illness treatment, is not so much "managing care" as "managing the benefit"! Too often, NAMI families tell us that managed care really means that they are rapidly managed out of all care and treatment. Their insurance benefit and access to care run out—but the severe and persistent mental illness continues.

NAMI families and consumers are a good "test case" for managed care in mental illness because we represent those most vulnerable to the problem of undertreatment and underrecognition.

A survey done by Johns Hopkins University in 1991 indicates that NAMI families bear unique burdens as they seek treatment and support for their mentally ill relatives. Over 1,400 NAMI members, in a representative sample drawn from across the country, responded to a 45-minute interview designed to clarify the needs of their mentally ill relative. Nearly 60% of NAMI members reported that their relative has schizophrenia. Bipolar disorder and severe recurrent depression affect 38% of NAMI members.

NAMI members are struggling with the impact of mental illness in an economy of cutback and downsizing. It is well understood in NAMI support groups that families are experts—they have become case managers by default. As the health care crisis deepens, our family members are picking up the pieces of their ill relatives' lives and filling in the gaps in care and coverage. Over 60% of NAMI members surveyed indicated that their ill relative's primary residence is the family home. This means that families are on duty 24 hours a day, 7 days a week, 365 days a year. We are, in fact, the "safety net" for our relatives who have mental illness. Mental health professionals have little appreciation of the enormous caregiving burden borne by families who have little training and support to rely on.

To be effective, managed care systems must ensure improved access, quality, and outcome for persons with mental illnesses.

There are a number of reasons why mentally ill individuals do badly in a managed care setting. Traditionally, health maintenance organizations have done a poor job of providing support services for persons with severe and persistent mental illnesses. Instead, they have designed policies that rapidly move people to the public sector. The public sector has become the "dumping ground" for the most seriously ill and disabled mental patients. It is good to remember that the state-based public system is itself beset by financial crisis. The safety net of public mental illness care is shredded. As NAMI pointed out in its 1992 study, "Criminalizing the Seriously Mentally Ill," we are seeing the most disabled mentally ill individuals who do not have access to needed treatment moving from the streets to the jails.

It is clear that by traditional standards, mentally ill individuals are viewed by health maintenance organizations and managed care companies as bad actuarial risks. Most mental health benefits are designed to focus on short-term treatment and crisis intervention. Although crisis intervention is clearly vital to persons experiencing episodes of psychosis, short-term treatment is insufficient for chronic illness. Most persons with severe and persistent mental illnesses also have poor physical health and have been high users of most medical services.

NAMI is also troubled by inadequate standards and safeguards for vulnerable patients and families who seek mental health treatment in a managed care setting. There is an enormous incentive to underrecognize and undertreat severe and persistent mental illnesses in a managed care environment. Even more troubling, most health maintenance organizations have little understanding of, or empathy for, mentally ill individuals and their medical psychiatric needs. Most programs seem designed to sort out those with "transitional mental health problems" from those with severe and persistent biologically based mental illnesses. The former group, sometimes called "the worried well," are generally well served by the limited benefits available under managed care programs. But those who are most in need of medical attention, most at risk for suicide, and most disabled by their illness are quickly routed to the public sector. Up to now, it appears that health maintenance organizations and managed care companies have controlled their spending on mental illness by "creaming"—that is, by serving those who need limited, short-term therapy while relying on the public sector to handle those who require more extensive and intensive treatment.

A look at what Medicaid history tells us makes it clear why this management strategy has become so popular in the managed care environment. Medicaid data tell us that severely mentally ill people are "costly" because they are prone to relapse and may be hospitalized repeatedly over a lifetime of illness. In fact, 35%–50% of all seriously mentally ill patients are rehospitalized within 6 months of discharge from initial hospitalization. Fully two-thirds of these readmissions occur within the first 3 months after initial discharge, and the average admission costs anywhere from $25,000 to $50,000.

These statistics underlie an important but often ignored management strategy: linkage and coordination between inpatient and outpatient care are essential for persons with serious and persistent mental illnesses. Without effective follow-up and ongoing aggressive case management, relapse and overutilization of hospital care become the striking signs of severe mental illnesses such as schizophrenia.

Another driver of costs is the problem of service fragmentation. Mentally ill individuals who are to be served in noninstitutional community settings must have access to more than medical care alone. Over 25 years of research on the Program of Assertive Community Treatment (PACT) indicates that even severely mentally ill people can do well in the community. Pioneered in Dane County, Wisconsin, this program has been proven effective in numerous sites across the country and around the world. Yet few managed care programs recognize and provide reimbursement for the full array of services required to maintain seriously mentally ill individuals in the community.

The PACT program provides for a continuous-treatment team that is permanently assigned to the mentally ill individual. The team is charged with providing a full range of medical, psychosocial, and rehabilitation services 7 days a week, 24 hours a day, for as long as the individual requires such service. There is a focus on providing treatment and teaching living skills in the home setting (e.g., a cooking lesson might be given in the patient's apartment) and on using community resources to build on the strengths of each patient (e.g., a patient might be taken to the YMCA or the YWCA to learn about recreational opportunities, or to the public library to see the books that help teach job-finding skills). There is also an assertive approach to case management. When someone misses an appointment or seems to be moving toward a relapse, the treatment team goes to the home of that individual to encourage and support appropriate medical attention. This aggressive approach to symptom reduction and prevention of relapse is designed to foster independent living and to improve the quality of life of both the patients and their families. PACT programs consistently reduce relapse and rehospitalization for severely mentally ill individuals.

The PACT program starts by recognizing a truth that seems to have eluded managed care company executives: there is a difference between mental health services useful for those with problems in living and mental illness services. Persons with severe mental illnesses must be understood and treated as a "special needs" population. NAMI families know that only a full array of treatment and services can meet their relatives' special needs and reduce overutilization of expensive crisis intervention and hospital care.

Psychiatrists and mental health professionals know that persons with severe and persistent mental illnesses do not respond well to brief therapy and crisis interventions alone. These patients have severe and recurring biologically based mental illnesses and must receive regular medical management as well as psychosocial rehabilitation services. They need a dedicated program to address all of their special needs. And they need this program to be available continually for as long as necessary. This care is not unlike the long-term care required to manage *any* chronic illness.

Much must be learned by providers before managed care companies can effectively provide good services for many seriously mentally ill people. Today in psychiatric care, we have the unique situation of the most severely ill and disabled patients generally receiving the fewest services, and often receiving those services from the persons least well trained to provide them. This imbalance is a function of reimbursement policies that NAMI families hope will change as the playing field is leveled in health care reform.

To meet the needs of severely mentally ill individuals, managed care executives must learn much more about efficacy of today's treatments for mental illness. Managed care providers need to recognize that individuals with serious mental illnesses require a fundamentally different kind of service than that traditionally offered by health maintenance organizations. It is also important to know that severely mentally ill people do not usually have a job; their disability is so great that they don't have a protective employer to intercede for them if benefits are threatened or to monitor for abuses. Sometimes, mentally ill individuals are resistant to accepting psychiatric treatment; they may need to be encouraged and supported in maintaining a lifelong treatment regimen. Because people with mental illnesses often have few support structures, family care and support are even more crucial.

For most NAMI members, managed care has represented a threat of undertreatment, inappropriate treatment, and denial of treatment. This situation need not exist in the future, but in too many cases it has surely existed in the past. In a health care reform environment, we have an opportunity to rethink our service paradigms. NAMI recommends that managed care companies start with the "customer"—that is, by listening and learning from consumers of mental illness services and their families. Families need to be seen as central to rehabilitation, recovery, and prevention of relapse for persons with severe and persistent mental illnesses. And increasingly, mentally ill persons themselves are seeking and demanding an active voice in the development of systems of care designed to meet their needs.

Yet NAMI families repeatedly tell us that although they have had literally dozens of interactions with treatment providers and managed care systems over a period of many years, their opinion is almost never sought. Almost never are the families recognized or respected for the role they play. Numerous studies have proven that recovery is significantly improved—that is, people get better faster—when caring, loving families assist in the planning, treatment, and caregiving. Families are likely to play a key role in stabilizing their relative if they are supported by professionals before discharge from the hospital and during any period of crisis or change. Family members also often maintain medical records over many years, providing a comprehensive picture of the history of their relative's illness and treatment. They know which medications work and which do not. They know what stressors cause relapse, and how quickly their loved one can move forward in a rehabilitation program. Yet family expertise often is discounted or denied.

Many consumers of mental illness services tell us that they are tired of being told that the big problem with "mental patients" is their passivity and lack of compliance. Perhaps the lack of follow-up with outpatient treatment regimens and the lack of participation in treatment programs will help providers recognize that many of these programs are patronizing and irrelevant. Why do managed care companies reimburse day treatment programs that teach adults to make macramé plant holders but fail to reimburse consumer-run clubhouse models or consumer-run drop-in centers, which many people find effective and empowering? When the customer is asked what kinds of services are wanted and needed, providers may begin to initiate new services.

Perhaps the worst outcome of many managed care programs for mental illness is the too rapid discharge of patients who are psychotic or suicidal. This cost-containment strategy is not only foolish but also tragic. In many cases, premature discharge means that the individual will turn up in a shelter, a jail, or an emergency room. But all too often the outcome is suicide. We must not permit managed care strategies to focus more on saving money than on saving lives.

> Mr. K. was a 23-year-old who had been increasingly troubled by severe depression for several years. He was hospitalized in a depressed and somewhat malnourished state after being gone from his family home for several weeks. After he spent 3 days in the hospital and new medication was prescribed, the managed care company moved to discharge Mr. K. Because the hospital staff recognized the fragility of Mr. K.'s condition, they provided care for him without secure reimbursement for an additional 3 days. But on day 6, Mr. K. was discharged. The in-hospital physician was supposed to link Mr. K. for aftercare through a social worker. Somehow, that connection was missed, and there was no follow-up in the days after Mr. K.'s discharge. Predictably enough, Mr. K. left his family home as he had in the past. Several days later, Mr. K.'s family learned that he had killed himself.

To NAMI families and mentally ill individuals, Mr. K.'s death is directly attributable to draconian managed care policies—policies carried out on a "one-size-fits-all" basis. Too many providers attempt to deal with symptoms and individual suffering using a benefit design that rations care in a way that is not rational.

As we move to a new environment of health care reform, it is imperative that executives in managed care and health maintenance organizations listen to mentally ill individuals and their families and learn from the bitter experiences of Ms. J. and Mr. K. It is possible and important to control runaway medical costs. But it is not necessary to do so at the cost of human lives. More must be done to match the intensity of treatment to the intensity of illness. More must be done to forge partnerships with mentally ill individuals and their families, to create connections between inpatient and outpatient settings, and to recognize that there are measures of success more important than the bottom line. The needs of the economy, even in these difficult times, cannot come before the needs of severely ill and uniquely vulnerable patients. To help improve the match between intensity of treatment and the intensity of illness, NAMI has taken steps to initiate a services research agenda focused on managed care and its impact on persons with severe mental illness and their families.

Section VI

Managing Care, Not Dollars

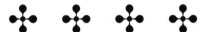

❖ 14 ❖

How Adversaries Can Become Allies

ROBERT K. SCHRETER, M.D.[*]
STEVEN S. SHARFSTEIN, M.D., M.P.A.[**]
CAROL A. SCHRETER, M.S.W., PH.D.[***]

This book is about the impact of managed care on mental health services. The advent of managed care is the result of the success in expanding and diversifying mental health care. Just 30 years ago there were essentially two choices—state mental hospitals for the many and psychoanalysis for the privileged few. Now there are a range of mental health care providers and a range of treatments. Health policy analysts talk about universal access to mental health care.

Both payers and clinicians are concerned about costs, but for different reasons. Payers watch the total cost—the bottom line. Clinicians focus on the individual. They see the allocation of resources affecting patients and those who cannot be treated for lack of insurance coverage.

Policymakers speak of managed care or managed competition as a

[*]Private practice in psychiatry, Baltimore, Maryland; Medical Director, Psych Services, Baltimore, Maryland; Assistant Professor of Psychiatry, Johns Hopkins Medical School, Baltimore, Maryland.
[**]Medical Director and Chief Executive Officer, The Sheppard and Enoch Pratt Hospital, Baltimore, Maryland; Clinical Professor of Psychiatry, University of Maryland Medical School, Baltimore, Maryland.
[***]Authors' editor and freelance writer on health and aging, based in Baltimore, Maryland.

solution to escalating health care costs. For many patients and family members, managed care represents a threat of undertreatment, inappropriate treatment, and denial of treatment. This book shows that managed care needs to be distinguished from managed costs. We do not know how to manage care. We are learning to manage costs. Managing care involves a focus on quality of care and outcomes. It is not yet possible because mental health professionals have not reached agreement on how to define and measure outcomes.

This book shows that managed care is not a solution, but a framework for a process. This process involves answering some very basic questions such as 1) how much money is needed, 2) where the money should go, 3) who should pay, 4) who should use mental health services, and 5) who should decide these questions.

Managed care is not a system, but a nonsystem. It involves different companies with different criteria. Mental health clinicians are mystified when distant reviewers say that care is not reimbursable ("not medically necessary") based on unpublished company criteria. Reviewers seem inconsistent in their decisions.

What is reimbursable? Why is this such a mystery? This crucial question is considered on a case-by-case basis. The question of reimbursement arises at the start of treatment and at multiple points along the way—because reimbursable care is being authorized in small pieces.

We believe that solving the cost problem must involve discussions among the different players. The number of players is increasing. There used to be three major players: the doctor, the patient, and the third-party insurer. Now there are six major players, including the cost-conscious employer, the managed care company, and the government. The speed of change is remarkable. Trained to be patient and thoughtful, mental health clinicians are ill equipped to provide guidance in this fast-paced environment.

To bring the focus back onto clinical care, this book has spotlighted the critical interaction between two of these players: the managed care reviewer and the mental health provider. In each chapter, a representative of the managed care industry has spoken, and then a clinician has spoken.

Readers may have found a repetition of identified problems and solutions. Do not consider this repetition a weakness. The editors consider it to be the strength of this book. These essays, written between February and May of 1993, provide a snapshot of the impact of managed costs on clinical practice. These essays from leaders in the field bring into sharp focus areas of disagreement and emerging agreement between clinicians and reviewers.

Certainly the contributors to this book were chosen for their moderate positions on managed mental health care. But even the editors were surprised to see the overlap of views. The adversarial posture that existed between managed care reviewers and providers is turning into a more cooperative effort. Both communities seem to be searching for quality, cost-effective psychiatric interventions—for a way to manage care, not just costs. The shared concerns and solutions represent a merging agreement not entirely predictable when this book was first conceived.

Areas of Adversity

This book has identified some critical problems with managed mental health care. Case vignettes have pointed out philosophical differences and how good theory can be ruined by inefficient procedures. The management of care can be an obstacle because of small issues—because of policies and procedures such as the following:

❖ A psychiatrist calling a managed care company for authorization must dictate the necessary information to a clerk who does not know how to spell the medical terminology.

❖ A provider must get care preauthorized by a managed care company located in Hawaii, six time zones away. Their workdays overlap only 2 hours a day.

❖ A managed care company is willing to authorize care, but does not have up-to-date information on the dollar value of care still available to the patient.

❖ A young couple with a 6-month-old child seeks counseling when their arguments lead to pushing, shoving, and potential violence. The managed care company authorizes just three outpatient visits and then, reluctantly, two more. The wife is eligible for 20 outpatient sessions a year; however, the managed care company prefers to reserve the remaining 15 sessions for future crises.

Such nuts-and-bolts situations echo critical themes voiced in many of these essays.

Who Will Be Treated? Who Will Be Excluded?

Some managed care companies now make their criteria for reimbursement public, helping to define what is considered "medically necessary." Making criteria public is essential and should be followed by discussion. The underlying values and philosophy should be refined based on feedback from care providers. It is clear that some clinicians, as managed care executives, are making more money by denying care than they ever made by providing care.

This book has highlighted some of the issues that await resolution. Clinicians are asking whether it is appropriate to hospitalize patients only if (and only as long as) they are dangerous to themselves and others. A 24-hour review and appeals process may be necessary. Timely decision making is crucial, both to controlling costs and to the therapeutic process. Clinicians think that a refusal to pay should involve a reviewer with the appropriate specialty training and an explanation about how the decision was reached.

In the march toward cost-effectiveness, less-impaired persons and those in need of preventive care are being excluded. Medicine in general is criticized for operating on a pathology model—for focusing on disease instead of prevention. Historically, preventive care has been a strength in mental health services. Now, people seeking preventive care are called the "worried well," and their treatment is not reimbursed. Instead, prevention deserves a significant percentage of the mental health dollar.

Disagreement About Clinical Interventions

Who makes the treatment decisions, and who will be accountable? What treatments will be funded, and for how many days?

Managed care reviewers say that denying payment is not the same as denying care. But clinicians and their patients disagree. Consider this situation. A suicidal, depressed patient is hospitalized. On the fifth day, the patient is deemed no longer suicidal. The reviewer says that care is no longer reimbursable. The clinician counters that discharge is premature.

Without insurance coverage, the patient is discharged—and commits suicide 4 days later. Who is responsible for this death and this decision? The courts are ambiguous about the accountability of the reviewer. But the treating clinician is accountable.

Disagreement often emerges around patient readiness for care at a level lower than acute hospitalization. Clinicians see that the boundaries between inpatient and outpatient care are now blurred. Treatment intensity and the place of delivery have been uncoupled. Both clinicians and managers must accept responsibility for developing a continuum of services, including group homes, partial hospitalization, and intensive outpatient care. However, these are unlikely to be developed unless reimbursement for such services is ensured.

Clinicians wonder whether chronic conditions will improve when they are treated as acute episodes. Short-term goals and treatments are now authorized for many patients for whom the underlying conditions are clearly lifelong issues. The goal of stabilization means that patients are not helped to reach their maximum potential. Employers want maximum productivity. Are they willing to settle for minimum productivity?

On the other hand, managers say that clinicians fail to recognize the difference between cost-effective and second-class care. Many managers firmly believe that short-term, issue-focused treatment is more likely to benefit *most patients*. Clinicians suspect that fraudulent abuses, unnecessary admissions, and unwarranted lengths of stay are a thing of the past. But managers assert that outdated professional training leads to treatment bias and that self-interest continues to affect treatment choice and duration.

Overall, regulators fault clinicians for focusing on the individual patient. They caution that integrated health systems will be responsible for huge populations of patients at fixed, negotiated rates. This situation will force clinical decision makers to shepherd scarce resources for huge numbers of lives.

How Can Administrative Costs Be Reduced so That There Is More Money for Patient Care?

The developing managed care scenario generates new costs. Clinicians find that dealing with managed care companies increases the time involved in treatment by about 20%. This time is not reimbursed. A managerial class of therapists are employed as reviewers at the managed care company. Up-to-date computer technologies are needed to track individual patient treatments and costs. Who will pay for these things? There are now up to three additional layers of profit taking: the national managed care firm, the local vendor, and the community-based multispecialty mental health group. They all incur costs and expect a profit for their efforts. This money is coming out of patient benefits.

Systemic Changes Require Changes in Clinician Training

Clinical roles are being redefined by a cost-benefit yardstick. Today's clinicians were trained in the biopsychosocial model, which values complexity and comprehensiveness without regard to cost. Clinicians are realizing that they need to balance the individual's welfare with the overall costs and benefits to society.

This balancing process is complex and should stimulate three separate training efforts. Treatment decisions are guided by a managerial class of reviewers, who may need special training. Practicing clinicians need retraining. At graduate schools and traineeships, future clinicians need instruction in the best possible use of a continuum of care. Who will bear the costs of such training?

At this point, most managed care companies will not even reimburse care provided by clinicians in training. Where contracts go to the lowest bidder, training facilities will never get contracts.

Becoming Allies

The areas of disagreement are substantial. Nevertheless, managed care executives and clinicians seem to agree on some broad and important issues in mental health care.

Cost Is a Legitimate Factor in Making Treatment Decisions

Managed care is here to stay. The worst is past. The hostility and confrontation of recent years seem to be leading to a time for frank discussion.

The process of external utilization review was painful. But providers are now joining cost-conscious networks. Some networks are assuming the financial risks and taking back clinical decision-making roles as they turn into accountable health plans.

Inpatient Psychiatric Stays Can Be Shorter

Inpatient care has been overinsured, and outpatient care has been underinsured. For both treatment and assessment, the duration of a hospital stay can be flexible, tailored to the situation and individual. There is nothing magical about 30 days. Aggressive efforts at hospital diversion and shortened lengths of stay have not, apparently, produced the vast number of catastrophes that some clinicians predicted.

A Continuum of Care Is Necessary and Desirable

Intermediate levels of care (i.e., treatment options less intense than the hospital stay and more intense than the weekly outpatient visit) are not new. However, they are now a fast-growing segment of the industry.

Practice Guidelines Are Needed

The review process will be much easier when practice guidelines are standardized. The managed care industry, the American Psychiatric Association, and other professional organizations are working on this. They hope that standardizing treatment procedures will make it easier to assess the quality of care provided.

But how broad or detailed should such guidelines be? For example, when a patient is admitted for suicidal depression, should the facility start antidepressant drugs immediately, or first observe the patient for 24 hours? Some managed care companies will not now pay for a day of observation. Others will. This is confusing for both providers and reviewers.

Outcome Studies Are Needed

Does mental health treatment work? Do patients get better? This is the critical issue as we move to the stage of managing care, not just costs. Both providers and managed care reviewers seem to agree that it is time to focus on patient outcomes.

Outcome research is expensive. But the main problem now is in determining what factors to measure. Customer satisfaction is only one element of quality. With psychiatric care, where the patient's judgment is often impaired, it may be important to include the family's perspective in measures of satisfaction. Managed care tends to focus on a patient's ability to perform normal activities of daily living unassisted.

Are clinicians to fight fires by treating only acute episodes? Clinicians used to seek greater benefit from mental health treatment. Their goal was improving the patient's quality of life or capacity to love and work. It is easier to measure days of work missed than performance on the job. People in distress commonly work harder and produce less. What about measures of overall health? Anxiety and depression are associated with higher use of other costly health services.

Mortality and frequency of readmission are already being tracked. But how do we measure morbidity? In terms of mental health, the percentage of a population with a diagnosable, treatable condition depends on the measures used. It is not yet clear how to measure severity of illness or the effectiveness of interventions.

Managed care companies hope that study of the utilization patterns of patients in their computerized files will lead to practice and quality guidelines. But depending on this readily available information does not conform to the scientific method. Such studies lack randomized control groups and controls for patient characteristics. Such studies are not prospective.

Managed mental health care as practiced today is fragmented and inefficient. Managing care involves more than managing costs. Providing quality care will require more dialogue between managed care executives and providers. This book, a chorus of voices of mental health industry leaders, is intended as a guide to the road ahead. In future discussions, patient care must be our indelible focus.

Index

*Page numbers printed in **boldface** type refer to figures.*

✥ A ✥

Abuse victims in inpatient care, 27–28

Access
importance of, in child and adolescent services, 79–80
importance of, in mental health and substance abuse services, 59–60
and quality-of-care guidelines, 182–183
role of managed care in improving, 204–205

Accountability, 6–7
and team services, 78

Accountable health plans
evolution of fee-for-service plans to, 3–8
need for, 7–8

Acute-care cases, 217
partial hospitalization for, 40–41

Acute-stabilization philosophy, 27–28

Adjunctive programs in child and adolescent services, 82–83

Administrative costs, need to reduce, 217–218

Adolescents. *See* Child and adolescent services

Aetna, 21

Agency for Health Care Policy and Research, 174

Alcohol. *See* Drug and alcohol abuse treatment

Alcoholics Anonymous (AA), 82, 89, 92, 160

American Academy of Child and Adolescent Psychiatry, 173, 174
"Outcomes and Treatment Efficacy Project," 75
practice parameters of, 74, 158

American Association for Partial Hospitalization, 34
on partial hospital program staffing, 38

American Hospital Association, 172

American Managed Care and Review Association, 173

American Medical Association
and development of practice guidelines, 165
and development of quality-of-care guidelines, 172
Principles of Medical Ethics, 194

American Psychiatric Association (APA), 115
and commercial review business, 176
and community service, 130
and development of practice guidelines, 153, 158, 163–164, 165, 166, 219
and ethical issues, 131, 194
and goal of standardized practice, 177–178
quality-of-care guidelines of, 170, 172, 179–180, 185

American Psych Management, 6

American Psychological Association
and marketing of managed care plan, 176
and quality-of-care-guidelines, 171, 172

American Psych Systems, 39–40
American Society of Addiction
    Medicine, 173
Assessment, role of psychologist in,
    129
Association of Medical
    Superintendents of American
    Institutions for the Insane, 163
Associations, role of psychologists
    in, 130
Attention-deficit hyperactivity
    disorder, exclusion from
    coverage, 63
Attitude, development of more
    cooperative, 19
Ayres, William, 75

✢ B ✢

Bayley, Nancy, 118
Benefit design strategy, 52
Bernfeld, Sigfried, 118
Biodyne, 19
Biopsychosocial assessments, 136
Biopsychosocial model for
    outpatient psychological
    services, 64
  psychosocial aspects of, 115
Blue Cross and Blue Shield
    Association, 172
Budman, S. H., 121

✢ C ✢

Carve-out contracts, 5–6, 198–199
Case management in lowering
    inpatient costs, 33
Case management companies, and
    need for cooperation between
    psychiatric hospitals, 30
Case review issues, in intermediate
    levels of care, 46–48
Catch-22 effect, 113

"Certificate of need" requirements,
    abolishment of, 12
Child and adolescent services
  abuse of inpatient hospitalization
    benefit for, 4
  clinician's view, 76–77
    dependence on support
      network, 78
    importance of access, 79–80
    importance of innovative
      programs, 80–84
    integrated network of
      self-managing teams, 78–79
    risks in, 77
  managed care view, 69–75
  role of partial hospital programs in
    meeting needs of, 39, 81–82
Children with Attention-Deficit
    Disorder (CH.A.D.D.), 83
CIGNA, 21
Civilian Health and Medical
    Program of the Uniformed
    Services (CHAMPUS),
    171–172, 180
Clinical interventions, disagreement
    about, 216–217
Clinical outcomes, in partial hospital
    programs, 39–40
Clinical standard, definition of, 170
Clinicians. See also Psychiatrists;
    Psychologists; Social workers
  need for cooperation in managed
    care, 213–20
  survival of, and outpatient
    services, 66–68
Clinician's view, xiii
  of child and adolescent services,
    76–77
  of drug and alcohol abuse
    treatment, 91–99
  of ethical issues under managed
    care, 195–200
  of inpatient services, 22

of intermediate levels of care, 41
of outpatient services, 60
of practice guidelines, 163–168
of psychiatrist's role, 108–116
of psychologist's role, 124–132
of quality-of-care guidelines,
    178–185
of social worker's role, 142–149
Clinician training, required changes
    in, 218
Community Mental Health Act, 142
Community mental health
    movement, xiii
    impact on psychiatry, 106
Community service, role of
    psychologists in, 130
Confidentiality
    as ethical issue, 199
    impact of managed care on, 24,
        113–114, 145–46
Conflict, in intermediate levels of
    care, 44–48
Conflicts of interest, 198
Constructive collaboration, 26
Continuing education, role of
    psychologists in, 131
Continuum of care
    in child and adolescent services, 73
    and ethical issues, 196–197
    hospital development of, 17
    need for, 219
    and utilization of provider
        networks, 114
Cost
    contributions by hospitals to
        problems of, 12–15
    as ethical issue, 192
    as factor in treatment decisions,
        64, 218–219
    need to reduce administrative,
        217–218
    and quality-of-care guidelines,
        183–184

Cost-versus-quality issue, conflicts
    over, 26–27
Creaming, 205–206
Crisis evaluation service, in partial
    hospital programs, 36
Criteria, problems with, in practice
    guidelines, 164–167
Cummings, N. A., 120, 121

✢ D ✢

Discharge, reforms in criteria for, 29
Double agentry, as ethical issue, 199
Drug and alcohol abuse treatment
    clinician's view, 91–99
    and employee assistance programs,
        136–41
    growth of programs for, 4
    managed care view, 85–91
DSM-III-R non-V code diagnosis,
    55–56, 58

✢ E ✢

Eating disorders, development of
    practice guidelines for,
    167–168
Economic incentives, as ethical
    issue, 199–200
Eddy, David, 166
Education Prevention Intervention
    Consultants (EPIC), 83–84
Efficiency in providing outpatient
    services, 64
"80/20" principle of management,
    54–55
Elwood, Paul, 176
Employee assistance programs
    (EAPs), 136–141
Employee psychologists, movement
    of, into management track, 128
Employers, education of, on need for
    mental health coverage, 30

Episodes of care, in outpatient treatment, 66
Ethical issues under managed care
clinician's view of, 195–200
managed care view of, 187–194
Ethical practice, role of psychologists in, 131–132
Excess hospital bed capacity, 12

✣ F ✣

Families of mentally ill patients, impact of managed care on, 25–26
Federal Employee Health Benefit Program, 170
Federal Employees Blue Cross Plan, 179
Fee-for-service plans, evolution of, to accountable health plans, 3–8
Feinstein, Alvan, 157
Focused outpatient treatment, 65
For-profit hospital chains, expansion into psychiatric and substance abuse care, 12, 93
Forward Plan for Health FY 1977–1981 (DHEW), 184–185
Four Winds Hospital, 18
Fraud and abuse in the hospital industry, 14
Full entitlement, 8
Functional outcome measures, importance of, 7

✣ G ✣

Gatekeeping function of managed care, 137
General practice of psychology, 120
Goal-oriented outpatient treatment, 65
Green Spring Health Services, 19
Group practice arrangements, trend toward, 104–105
Group treatment, 127

✣ H ✣

Health care
goals of, 181
increases in costs, 3
Health care reform
effect of, on managed care, 20–22
need for, 3–4, 31
and quality-of-care guidelines, 184–185
reasons for current interest in, 181–182
Health Insurance Association of America, 172
Health Maintenance Organization Act of 1973, 60
Health maintenance organizations (HMOs)
cost expectations of, 198
creaming policies in providing mental health coverage, 205–206
drug and alcohol abuse treatment services in, 97
and ethical issues, 195, 198
in providing child and adolescent services, 77, 81
in providing intermediate levels of care, 44
in providing outpatient care, 56
social worker involvement with, 136, 137
Health Plan Purchasing Cooperatives, 40
Hospitals. *See also* Partial hospital programs (PHPs)
contributions by, to problem of cost versus quality, 12–15
delays in technology transmission, 14–15
excess hospital bed capacity, 12, 23
fixed lengths of stay, 13
fraud and abuse, 14

overreliance on inpatient care as preferred treatment modality, 12–13
profit motive, 13–14

✛ I ✛

Indemnity insurance system, choices in, 53
Independent practice association–health maintenance organizations (IPA-HMOs), for outpatient services, 56, 58
Individualization of treatment, 18
In-home health care, 31
Inpatient services
abuse of hospitalization benefit for, 4
clinician's view, 22–23
finding solutions, 28–30
impact on staff, patients, and families, 23–26
major areas of conflict, 26–28
differentiating partial hospital programs from, 37–38
drug and alcohol abuse treatment, 83–86, 93–95
impact of managed care on, 33, 34, **34**
length of stays in, 29, 219
managed care view, 11–22
changes in the hospital industry, 17–19
changes in the managed care industry, 19–20
future, 20–22
hospital contributions to problem of cost versus quality, 12–15
problems in managed care industry, 15–17
as preferred treatment modality, 12–13, 32, 76
rise in costs of, 33

society's view of, 23
Institute of Medicine report, 96
Insurance companies
under indemnity system, 53, 57
and profit motive, 14
and reimbursement for drug and alcohol abuse treatment, 85
and reimbursement for mental health services, 32–33, 199–200
and use of practice guidelines, 167–168
and use of quality-of-care guidelines, 172
InterCare, 77
interdisciplinary collaboration, role of psychologists in, 131
Intermediate levels of care
clinician's view, 41–42
areas of stress and conflict, 44–48
future directions, 49
institutional capacity to cope with managed care, 42–43
managed care's impact, 43–44
managed care view, 31–32
patient satisfaction and clinical outcomes, 39–40
role for freestanding partial hospital programs, 32–36
treatment in partial hospital programs, 36–39
as treatment of choice for most acute-care cases, 40–41
Intervention Project for Nurses, 147

✛ J ✛

Joint Commission on Accreditation of Healthcare Organizations, on partial hospital program staffing, 38

❖ K ❖

Kaiser Health Plans, 56
Karasu, Byram, 163

❖ L ❖

Lengths of stay. *See also* Utilization
    review
    curtailing, and cost savings, 29
    fixed, 13
    movement to shorter, 18
    need for flexibility in, 219
    utilization review focus on, 78–79

❖ M ❖

Malpractice litigation crisis, 13
Managed care
    and cooperation with clinicians in,
        213–220
    definition of, 41–42
    ethical issues under
        clinician's view, 195–200
        managed care view, 187–194
    evolution of, xiii
    impact on confidentiality, 24,
        113–114, 145–146
    impact on intermediate levels of
        care, 43–44
    and inpatient costs, 33, 34, **34**
    and mental illness, 203–210
    utilization review in, 4–5
Managed care companies
    conflict between psychiatric
        hospitals and, 11
    creaming policies in providing
        mental health coverage,
        205–206
    and 80/20 principle of
        management, 54
    employment of former mental
        health clinicians by, 55

hospital systems as, 17–18
    and prevention of overutilization
        of services, 42
    profit motive in, 65
    and use of provider contracts,
        53–54
Managed care view
    of child and adolescent services,
        69–75
    of drug and alcohol abuse
        treatment, 85–91
    of ethical issues under managed
        care, 187–194
    of inpatient services, 11–22
    of intermediate levels of care, 31
    of outpatient services, 51–54
    of practice guidelines, 153–162
    of psychiatrist's role, 103–108
    of psychologist's role, 117–123
    of quality-of-care guidelines,
        169–178
    of social worker's role, 135–141
Managed competition, 7, 26, 59
Management Health Networks, 6
Management of care, drug and
    alcohol abuse treatment in,
    97–98
Mateer, Florence, 118
MCC Behavioral Care, 137
    and publication of practice
        guidelines, 154–162
Medicaid, and coverage of mentally
    ill, 206
Medicare
    cost-containment provisions of,
        178–179
    and utilization review, 179
Menninger, William, 117
Menninger, C. F., Memorial Hospital
    impact of managed care at, 23–26
    major areas of conflict at, 26–28
Mental health care costs, increases
    in, 3–4

Mental health professionals,
continuing and evolving roles
of, 176–177
Mental health services
development of quality-of-care
guidelines in, 170–174
development of two-class system
in outpatient services,
63–64
functional outcome measures for,
7
historical development of, xiii
need for reforms in, 3–4
role of partial hospital programs
in, 32–41
Mental illness, and managed care,
203–210
Mental Retardation Facilities and
Community Mental Health
Center Construction Act (1963),
32
Minnesota model of
abstinence-oriented addiction
treatment, 92, 95

✛ N ✛

National Alliance for the Mentally Ill
(NAMI), and managed care,
204–210
National Association of Insurance
Commissioners, 173
National Association of
Manufacturers, 172
National Association of Social
Workers, 141
National Mental Health Leadership
Forum, 177
National Register of Health Care
Providers in Psychology, 125
Nurses, role of, in utilization review,
4, 5

✛ O ✛

Oregon Health Decisions, 175
Outcomes and Treatment Efficacy
Project (AACAP), 75
Outcome focused on dysfunction, in
outpatient treatment, 66
Outcome focused on stabilization, in
outpatient treatment, 66
Outcomes management
functional measures in, 7
and quality-of-care guidelines,
174–177
Outcome studies, need for, 219–220
Outpatient services
clinician's view, 60
clinicians in, 66–68
patients in, 60–64
providers in, 64–65
treatment, 65–66
defining, 54
differentiating partial hospital
programs from, 37–38
managed care view, 51–54
considerations in, 55–56
future of, 59–60
managed care strategies in,
56–59
managed care thinking in, 54–55
Overutilization, role of managed care
in prevention of, 42

✛ P ✛

Paperwork, involvement of
psychiatrists in, 112
Paradigm shifts, need for, 6–7
Parents of Teens Addicted to Drugs
and Alcohol (POTADA), 83
Partial hospital programs (PHPs), 31
in child and adolescent services,
39, 81–82
crisis evaluation service in, 36

PHPs *(continued)*
  differentiating from outpatient and
    inpatient treatment, 37–38
  distinction between freestanding
    and hospital-based, 33–36
  evolution of new role for, 32–36
  financial benefits of, 33
  patient criteria for, 36–37
  and patient satisfaction and
    clinical outcomes, 39–40
  programming at, 38–39
  staffing of, 38
  as treatment of choice for most
    acute-care cases, 40–41
Patients
  appropriateness of partial hospital
    programs for, 36–37
  bill of rights for, 122
  concern over premature discharge
    of, 24–25, 209, 217
  impact of managed care on, 24–25
  in outpatient services, 60–64
  satisfaction of, and clinical
    outcomes, in partial hospital
    programs, 39–40
  stealing of, as ethical issue, 199
Peer review
  development of national program
    for, 171–172
  and inpatient stays, 23
Person-in-environment perspective,
  142–143
PHPs. *See* Partial hospital programs
  (PHPs)
Physician involvement, increased, 19
Pit-stop therapy, 115
Political involvement, role of
  psychologists in, 130
Posthospital environment, 28
PRACTICE acronym model,
  128–132
Practice guidelines
  clinician's view of, 163–168

managed care view of, 153–162
  need for, 219
  problems with current criteria,
    164–167
  use and misuse of, 167–168
Preferred Health, 6, 18
Preferred provider networks,
  development of, 20
Preferred provider organizations
  (PPOs), 56
  in child and adolescent services, 72
  cost expectations of, 198
  and ethical issues, 195, 198
  and utilization review, 57–58
Preferred treatment modality,
  overreliance on inpatient care as,
  12–13
Prescriptive outpatient treatment, 66
Prime provider, 119
Private practitioners, and patient
  referrals, 127–128
Professional autonomy, erosion of,
  126
Profit motive, 13–14
Programming, in partial hospital
  programs, 38–39
Program of Assertive Community
  Treatment (PACT), 206–207
Provider discounts, in lowering
  inpatient costs, 33
Provider networks, utilization of, and
  continuity of care, 114
Providers in outpatient services,
  64–65
Psychiatric hospitals
  conflict between managed care
    companies, 11
  movement to shorten lengths of
    stay, 18
  and need for cooperation between
    case management companies,
    30
  profit motive of, 13–14

Psychiatrists
  clinician's view of role of, 108–116
  exodus of, from community mental
    health marketplace, 106
  involvement in utilization review, 19
  managed care view of role of,
    103–108
  marketing efforts of, 53, 105–106,
    115
  reestablishment of, as medical
    directors, 119
  and utilization review, 24
  view of managed care by, 53
Psychodiagnosis, 127
Psychologists
  clinician's view of role of, 124–132
  erosion of professional autonomy,
    126
  functions of, 127–128
  managed care view of role of,
    117–123
  marketing efforts of, 53
  and patient referrals, 127–128
  and PRACTICE acronym model,
    128–132
  role expectations in, 126
Psychology, evolution of profession,
    117–118
Psychopharmacology
  revolution in, 118–119
  role of psychiatrist in, 106, 109
Psychotherapy
  role of psychiatrist in, 106–110
  role of psychologist in, 118–122,
    129
Public criteria, in managed care, 19

❖ Q ❖

Quality, contributions by hospitals to
    problem of cost versus, 12–15
Quality assurance activities, and
    mental health professionals, 53

Quality-of-care guidelines, 183
  access in, 182–183
  clinician's view of, 178–185
  cost in, 183–184
  development of in current mental
    health services, 170–174
  explicit, 169–170
  and health care reform, 184–185
  implicit, 170
  managed care view of, 53, 169–178
  and outcome management,
    174–177
  for partial hospital programs, 39–40
  quality in, 183
  and standardized practice, 177–178

❖ R ❖

Reik, Theodore, 118
Research
  need for outcome studies in,
    219–220
  politicization of models and data,
    175
  role of psychologist in, 129
Retained providers, 119–120
Review criteria, secret, 15
Review personnel, inappropriate
    credentials of, 15–16
Risk-sharing arrangements, 198

❖ S ❖

Scheduling, in partial hospital
    programs, 38
School-based services, in child and
    adolescent services, 83–84
Self-managing teams, in child and
    adolescent services, 78–79
Service delivery, fragmentation of,
    4
Short-term outpatient treatment, 65,
    217

Social Security Amendments of
    1972, 179
Social work administrators, in
    managed mental health care
    systems, 140
Social workers
    clinician's view of role of, 142–149
    managed care view of role of,
        135–141
    role of, in utilization review, 5
Staff, impact of managed care on,
    23–24
Staffing levels, in partial hospital
    programs, 38
Standardized practice, and quality-
    of-care guidelines, 177–178
Step-down care, 32, 35, 36
Stress, in intermediate levels of care,
    44–48
Structural problems, in intermediate
    levels of care, 44–46
Substance abuse inpatient programs
    and fixed lengths of stay, 13
    growth of, 4
    and individualization of treatment,
        18
    and malpractice crisis, 13
    movement to shorten lengths of
        stay, 18
    profit motive of, 13–14
Suicide, and early discharge, 209,
    217
Supplementary intensive programs,
    in child and adolescent services,
    80–84
Support network, children and
    adolescent dependence on, 78
System of care, accountability of, 7–8

❖ T ❖

Teaching, role of psychologists in,
    130

Team approach
    in child and adolescent services,
        78–79
    in drug and alcohol abuse
        treatment, 96
Technology transmission, delays in,
    14–15
Telephone utilization review, 72, 76,
    78, 119, 195
Third-party reimbursement for
    mental health services, 32–33
Three-way relationship (managed
    care triangle), **144**
Treatment, in outpatient services,
    65–66
Treatment decisions, cost as factor
    in, 218–219
Treatment research, effect of, on
    managed care, 96–97
23-hour observation, in child and
    adolescent services, 80

❖ U ❖

Underbidding
    as problem with carve-out
        contracts, 6
    role of accountable health plan in
        preventing, 8
Undertreatment and managed care,
    208
Underutilization, 127
United Auto Workers, 172
United Health Care, 21
U.S. Behavioral Health, 6
Universal access, and quality-of-care
    guidelines, 182–183
Utilization review
    in child and adolescent services, 73
    conflict between criteria used for,
        and medical necessity, 27
    and development of more
        cooperative attitude, 19

development of public criteria for, 19

in drug and alcohol abuse treatment, 89–91

establishing practice guidelines for, 29

and inappropriate credentials of new personnel, 15–16

involvement of physicians in, 19

in managed care, 4–5

and Medicare, 179

and need to redefine role of reviewer, 24, 29–30

and preferred practice organizations, 57–58

rationing in, for outpatient services, 59

secret criteria in, 15

steps in, for outpatient services, 56–57

telephone, 72, 76, 78, 119, 195

Utilization Review Accreditation Commission, 20, 172

Utilization Review Accreditation Council (URAC), on secret criteria, 166

✣ V ✣

VandenBos, G. R., 120

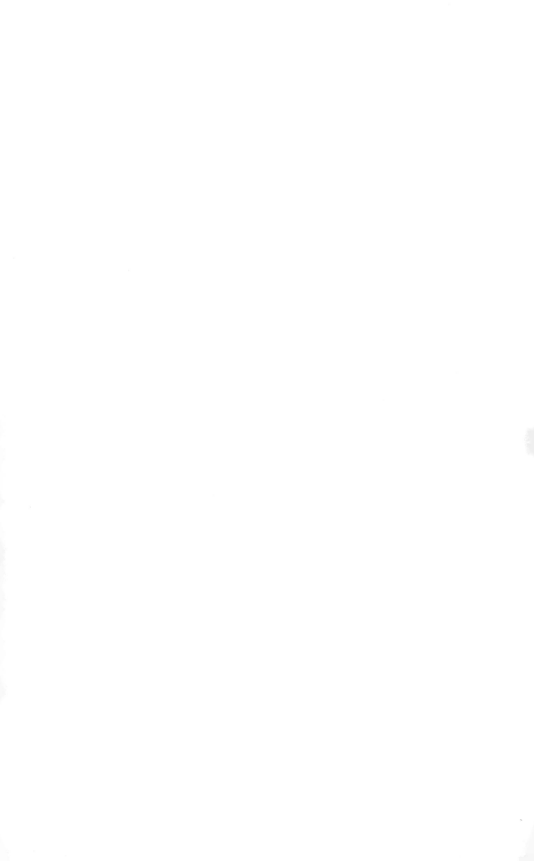